Current Topics in Environmental Health and Preventive Medicine

Series Editor:

Takemi Otsuki
Kurashiki, Japan

Current Topics in Environmental Health and Preventive Medicine, published in partnership with the Japanese Society of Hygiene, is designed to deliver well written volumes authored by experts from around the globe, covering the prevention and environmental health related to medical, biological, molecular biological, genetic, physical, psychosocial, chemical, and other environmental factors. The series will be a valuable resource to both new and established researchers, as well as students who are seeking comprehensive information on environmental health and health promotion.

More information about this series at http://www.springer.com/series/13556

Fumihiro Sata • Hideoki Fukuoka
Mark Hanson
Editors

Pre-emptive Medicine: Public Health Aspects of Developmental Origins of Health and Disease

Springer

Editors
Fumihiro Sata
Chuo University Health Center
Tokyo
Japan

Hideoki Fukuoka
Waseda University
Tokyo
Japan

Mark Hanson
University of Southampton
Academic Unit of Human Development
& Health
Southampton
UK

ISSN 2364-8333 ISSN 2364-8341 (electronic)
Current Topics in Environmental Health and Preventive Medicine
ISBN 978-981-13-2193-1 ISBN 978-981-13-2194-8 (eBook)
https://doi.org/10.1007/978-981-13-2194-8

Library of Congress Control Number: 2018961839

This Springer imprint is published by the registered company Springer Nature Singapore Pte Ltd.
The registered company address is: 152 Beach Road, #21-01/04 Gateway East, Singapore 189721, Singapore

Foreword

Noncommunicable diseases (NCDs), such as cardiovascular diseases, diabetes mellitus, and obesity, are becoming worldwide health and economic burden because of an increasing aged population both in developed and developing countries. It is imperative, therefore, to develop more effective means for preventing a variety of age-associated NCDs.

Most of NCDs are considered to develop through interplays between genetic make-up and environmental factors. Recent progress in genomics, especially genome-wide association studies (GWAS), has identified numerous variants associated with NCDs. For example, in essential hypertension and type 2 diabetes mellitus, more than 90 genetic variants have been reported to be associated with each of diseases. Such variants could explain, however, only a part of heritability of such diseases because effect sizes of each variant are very small. This is the case in many other NCDs that have been studied by the GWAS and is called "missing heritability."

Since most variants discovered by GWAS are located in the DNase 1 hypersensitive sites of the genome, not in protein-coding regions but in promoter or enhancer regions. This suggests that altered gene expression may be of importance for developing NCDs and that environmental factors play at least partly important roles.

Numerous epidemiological and experimental studies in the past decades have shown that adverse environment in fetal or early neonatal periods, such as malnutrition, environmental chemicals, and stress, is associated with increased prevalence of NCDs in later life. This concept is now called Developmental Origins of Health and Disease (DOHaD), since early environment may affect both health and diseases in later life. The underlying mechanism which explains the long-lasting effect throughout life course is thought to be epigenetic changes, which have been demonstrated by many animal experiments and some human studies. Some epigenetic changes are now considered to be potentially transmitted to several generations and are possibly related to the enormous increases of obesity worldwide.

Prevention of NCDs in adulthood has been an important issue in public health for a long time. The approach used to be population-based, identifying risk factors in cohort studies and managing them focusing on adult lifestyle. There has been less interest in personalized or precision medicine approach which is based on not only genomics but also environmental factors from the fetal life. In the era of precision medicine, pre-emptive medicine is required, which aims for personalized preventive medicine, taking genetics, epigenetics, environmental factors from fetal life, and potential biomarkers into account. The goal of pre-emptive medicine is to predict latent disease process with high probability and do early intervention in order to prevent disease onset. For this goal, we need more studies on genomics and epigenetics of NCDs, biomarkers for predicting latent disease process, and personal health data of each individual from various stages of life course. A strategic approach is required to establish new public health in the era of pre-emptive medicine.

Kyoto University, Kyoto, Japan Hiroo Imura

Preface

It is our great pleasure to publish the Springer book entitled "*Pre-emptive Medicine: Public Health Aspects of Developmental Origins of Health and Disease.*" This book is one of the official series of the Japanese Society for Hygiene, "Current Topics in Environmental Health and Preventive Medicine."

The concept of Developmental Origins of Health and Disease (DOHaD) was based on a series of epidemiological studies that were conducted by David J. Barker and his colleagues in Southampton, UK, in the 1980s, which linked the state of health and causes of death in the later stages of life to fetal development, assessed by birth weight. Barker's observations followed those of others who had shown long-term effects of aspects of the developmental environment, and made it clear that the risk of noncommunicable diseases (NCDs) in particular needed to be considered across the whole life course, and even across generations. This research field became known as the fetal origins of adult disease. Barker's observations were soon confirmed in a range of other longitudinal cohorts in both developed and developing countries, and by a range of experimental and clinical studies. From the outset, researchers focused on the effects of fetal undernutrition in initiating the trajectory of later NCD risk, especially if overconsumption of poor quality processed foods nutrition followed with rapid growth and obesity in early childhood. Other factors affecting fetal development including smoking, environmental chemicals, and maternal obesity were also shown to have long-term effects on later NCD risk. In the early years of this millennium, it became clear that the factors which could affect development, with long-term consequences, operated even during early embryonic life and continued through childhood development. Moreover, it became clear that these processes produced graded effects on normal developmental plasticity rather than inducing pathological changes, thus affecting later health as well as patterns of disease. The research field was therefore renamed the Developmental Origins of Health and Disease (DOHaD). The DOHaD concept has become widely known among multidisciplinary researchers. There is an International DOHaD Society, with very active regional chapters in many countries, including Japan. There is also a widely cited journal, *J. DOHaD*. DOHaD research has led to many new collaborations and large-scale studies involving networks and consortia, data integration, and meta-analysis of results. Analytical techniques, of genomes, epigenomes, and recently metagenomes, to incorporate the influence of effects on the microbiome, have dramatically advanced the understanding of the mechanisms underlying DOHaD and are leading to the discovery of novel early life biomarkers of later NCD risk. Data science has been developed to analyze the big data obtained and to coordinate the collection and analysis of biobanked samples. DOHaD-related papers have increased in number dramatically, and the DOHaD concept becomes more and more refined.

From the outset, DOHaD research has offered the prospect of early detection of individuals or populations at particular risk of later NCDs, for example those born with low birth weight or in countries undergoing rapid socio-economic and nutritional transitions. This might lead to the design of preventive measures to reduce such risk. This agenda has never been more important, as over 70% of deaths globally every year are due to NCDs, and about 80% of these deaths occur in low-middle income countries. Thus the concept of DOHaD has entered a new era in conjunction with a new personalized medical paradigm of pre-emptive medicine at the preventative or preclinical stage and precision medicine at the clinical stage. This is the theme of this volume.

We hope that this book will help a wide range of readers to understand and apply this new extended concept of DOHaD.

Tokyo, Japan Fumihiro Sata
Tokyo, Japan Hideoki Fukuoka
Southampton, UK Mark Hanson

Contents

Part I
General Remarks

Chapter 1
Maternal Exposure to Environmental Chemicals and Health Outcomes Later in Life

Chiharu Tohyama

Abstract The developmental origins of health and disease (DOHaD) paradigm, which was first presented as the Barker hypothesis, has been widely accepted in a variety of medical disciplines, ranging from public health to internal medicine, nutritional sciences, gynecology, pediatrics, and environmental health. Prenatal exposure to industrial chemicals at low doses has been shown to have a critical window during gestation and induce abnormalities later in life following a definite latent period. Such exposure scenarios can now be considered as a critical component that may act as initiating or modifying factors for health and disease status later in life and support the DOHaD paradigm. Exogenous chemicals include methylmercury, pesticides (organophosphates and neonicotinoids), tobacco, polychlorinated biphenyls and dioxins, and diethylstilbestrol, and their late-onset health outcomes include cancers and neurocognitive behavioral abnormalities. In order to understand the DOHaD paradigm, attention needs to be drawn to chemical exposure during the early life stages. Subtle alterations in developmental neurotoxicity that can only be detected by cutting-edge technology using a hypothesis-driven approach are discussed in the present study.

Keywords Chemical exposure · Dioxins · Environmental endocrine disruptors · Industrial chemicals · Methylmercury · Pesticides

---

C. Tohyama
Health, Environment, Science, and Technology International Consulting, Tokyo, Japan

Faculty of Medicine, University of Tsukuba, Tsukuba, Ibaraki, Japan

The University of Tokyo, Tokyo, Japan
e-mail: tohyama.chiharu@md.tsukuba.ac.jp

F. Sata et al. (eds.), *Pre-emptive Medicine: Public Health Aspects of Developmental Origins of Health and Disease*, Current Topics in Environmental Health and Preventive Medicine, https://doi.org/10.1007/978-981-13-2194-8_1

Abbreviations

ADI	Allowable daily intake
AhR	Aryl hydrocarbon receptor
AVPV	Anteroventral periventricular nucleus
BPA	Bisphenol A
CPF	Chlorpyrifos
DES	Diethylstilbestrol
DL	Dioxin-like
DOHaD	Developmental origins of health and disease
EDCs	Endocrine-disrupting chemicals
FOAD	Fetal origins of adult disease
JECFA	Joint FAO/WHO Expert Committee on Food Additives
MPOA	Medial preoptic area
nAChR	Nicotinic acetylcholine receptor
PCB	Polychlorinated biphenyl
PCDD	Polychlorinated dibenzo-*p*-dioxin
PCDF	Polychlorinated dibenzofuran
TCDD	2,3,7,8-tetrachlorodibenzo-*p*-dioxin

1.1 Introduction

Human health status is governed by predisposing factors determined by the genome of each individual, as well as by homeostatic regulation of the human body. Predisposition can develop during the evolution processes over a very long period of time, but it can be modulated in response to environmental stimuli, possibly by epigenetic mechanisms, and may be inherited by subsequent generations. Genetic factors were historically believed to play predominant roles in the etiology of chronic diseases, including cancers, cardiovascular disease, and type 2 diabetes mellitus, whereas lifestyle, including high-calorie diet, low level of physical activity, high-salt intake, tobacco, and alcohol, is now considered to significantly contribute to the incidence of these diseases [1]. The etiology of these diseases was challenged by the late Sir David Barker and his associates, who reported a number of epidemiologic studies describing that poor nutritional status during pregnancy is associated with increased rates of coronary heart disease, stroke, type 2 diabetes mellitus, adiposity, the metabolic syndrome, and osteoporosis in adult life [2, 3]. They proposed the "thrifty phenotype" hypothesis, stating that poor nutritional status in fetal and early infant life is detrimental to the development and function of the individuals' organism, predisposing them to the development of adult chronic diseases. This theory indicates that causal factors of adult-onset diseases may exist during early life, which lead to alteration of health status and disease phenotypes. With a greater number of observations that support the Barker theory by epidemiologic and clinical studies as well as laboratory animal studies, the term "Barker theory" was renamed FOAD (fetal origins of adult disease) and subsequently to DOHaD to recognize and broaden the concept that perinatal environment can shape both health and disease in resulting offspring [4]. Readers are suggested to refer to other articles in this book.

Because major health outcomes on which the DOHaD paradigm relies were lifestyle-related diseases, it was natural that the majority of researchers who led the study of the DOHaD paradigm at the initial stage were clinical or public health oriented and nutritional status was intensively investigated as a main environmental factor. However, researchers in the field of environmental health and toxicology who have been studying environmental pollutants as well as endocrine-disrupting chemicals (EDCs) realized that some of the important properties of these chemicals, such as late-onset toxicity, critical window, and latency, could have commonalities, although not entirely, with the DOHaD paradigm.

Until the late 1990s, the majority of scientific concerns on the possible impacts of environmental pollutants on public health have been directed to the occurrence of catastrophic diseases which occurred in various parts of the world. These include *Minamata* disease, *itai-itai* disease, chronic obstructive pulmonary diseases from air pollution, dioxin, and PCB-induced poisoning, chronic arsenic poisoning, and various types of cancers caused by exposure to asbestos, chromium, and other chemicals. In addition, toxicological research became institutionalized in the USA in response to public concern about cancer and acute mortality [5]. Little attention was paid to pesticides and industrial synthetic chemicals that have adverse effects on endocrine function. Incidentally, since the late 1990s, environmental chemicals that may act as "environmental estrogens" have gained increasing attention of researchers in toxicology, endocrinology and developmental biology, and epidemiology. In the late 1990s, the term "environmental hormones" was coined and used in official governmental documents and also used by Japanese media for some time. However, the use of this term has now been discontinued in official documents due to possible imprecise interpretations.

Scientists as well as stakeholders were challenged to hypothesize that humans and wildlife species have suffered adverse health effects after exposure to endocrine-disrupting chemicals (EDCs). The book, entitled *Our Stolen Future* by Colborn and associates [6], has become a milestone in research on the health of humans and wildlife. EDCs is defined as "an exogenous substance or mixture that alters function(s) of the endocrine system and consequently causes adverse health effects in an intact organism, or its progeny, or (sub) populations. A potential endocrine disruptor is an exogenous substance or mixture that possesses properties that might be expected to lead to endocrine disruption in an intact organism, or its progeny, or (sub) populations" [7]. In particular, the mode of action of EDCs is unique. Low-dose exposure to EDCs during early life (gestation and lactation periods) does not exert overt toxicity in mothers or offspring; there is often a critical window in gestational or neonatal periods. However, the latency period, between chemical exposure and the onset of symptoms later in life, is a premise of the DOHaD paradigm, but not necessarily for the mode of action of the EDCs.

1.2 Chemical Exposure and the DOHaD Paradigm

To examine when the "DOHaD" paradigm was intentionally internalized in the research on chemical exposure, in this review, I surveyed literature on Medline. A PubMed search using the term "DOHaD" in "all fields" yielded 269 papers as of April 21, 2017. The first paper that had the term "DOHaD" was published in 2005 [8]. When the terms "DOHaD" and "chemical" were searched together in "all fields," only 16 papers were found. A paper by Grun and Blumberg [9] specifically described an obesogen concept of chemicals, such as tributyltin, in the context of DOHaD. Bezek's short review [10] mentions chemical exposure in the context in DOHaD, but there is no detailed discussion. In a conference statement [11], the importance of research on the effects of prenatal and early postnatal exposure to chemical agents and their sustained effects on the individual throughout the lifespan was emphasized, and this concept was developed as the DOHaD paradigm. A review article by Rosenfeld [12] may be the first to comprehensively place chemical exposures in the DOHaD paradigm. In this review article, however, the endpoint of environmental chemical exposure was focused on an association of sex dimorphic responses of zygotes and conceptuses in response to exposure to EDCs, with neurobehavioral changes later in life as a DOHaD outcome.

Recently, Heindel and associates [13] reported a review article, based on their extensive survey of original papers in environmental epidemiology with regard to the DOHaD paradigm. The authors reviewed 2675 publications in environmental epidemiology and 425 publications published by the end of year 2014. They selected papers with contents essentially related to the DOHaD paradigm, or proof of concept approach, even if there was no mention on DOHaD in a given paper. The papers examined were original research in humans that examined the association between prenatal and/or early childhood exposures (up to 8 years old) to environmental chemicals and adverse health outcomes later in life. Based on their analysis, these papers dealt with perinatal exposure to 60 different chemicals (excluding tobacco, alcohol, and pharmaceuticals but including diethylstilbestrol as a prototypical chemical for the proof of concept) to the health effects later in life [13]. By a trend analysis of health outcomes, DOHaD epidemiology publications on adverse health outcomes are related to neurological/cognitive outcomes (n = 211 publications), followed by cancer (n = 59), respiratory (n = 50), metabolic outcomes including obesity (n = 35), reproductive health (n = 31), immune disorders (n = 29), endocrine (n = 22), and cardiovascular dysfunctions (n = 12) with less than 10 publications each focusing on the skin, musculoskeletal, visual problems, gastrointestinal, and liver. This review article claims that many papers on environmental chemical exposure that were published before the emergence of the Barker theory or DOHaD paradigm described phenomena that could still be explained by the DOHaD paradigm. Whether each paper cited in this review appropriately represents a DOHaD paradigm from the chemical exposure point of view should be evaluated by readers. It should be pointed out that the dataset of all the selected literature which is available to readers might be useful as a common platform for the literature survey on the DOHaD and chemical exposure research.

To sum up the two independent results on the literature surveys as described above, the DOHaD paradigm conceived by unique observations on poor nutritional status during early life was also influenced by environmental chemical exposure during this period. The influence of chemical exposure opened up a new avenue of research field in the context of the DOHaD paradigm. Since the majority of papers on chemical exposure-related DOHaD tend to deal with neurological/cognitive outcomes and cancer [13], this review mainly describes these types of disorders.

1.3 A Wide Spectrum of Health Outcomes by Chemical Exposure

The life of mammals, including humans, is regulated to maintain homeostasis in response to environmental stress. However, when the degree of stress, such as dose of a chemical, overwhelms the physiological capacity, homeostasis is disrupted, and abnormal signs and symptoms manifest. In case of chemical exposure, there are many examples in which the exposure level and timing of a chemical can induce severe systemic abnormalities. In the context of the DOHaD paradigm, such cases may represent an extreme end of the spectrum of abnormalities.

A prototypical example is *Minamata* disease, caused by methylmercury poisoning in Japan. The officially certified year of outbreak of this human tragedy was 1956. Many people living around *Minamata* Bay have been suffering from the effects of this chemical for several decades after exposure. Humans are protected from xenobiotic chemicals by barrier systems in the body. The most well-known barrier system is the blood-brain barrier, which is composed of a complex structure of astrocytes and unfenestrated endothelial cells in the capillaries. Another barrier system is the fetoplacental barrier, in which maternal and fetal circulation are separate and do not mix. However, these barrier systems are overwhelmed by excessive exposure to methylmercury. The inability of these barrier systems and the presence of a critical window of vulnerability were shown in *Minamata* disease. Methylmercury, a lipophilic low molecular weight chemical, can be easily transferred through the fetoplacental barrier and also through the blood-brain barrier even in adults. When pregnant women regularly ate heavily contaminated fish, methylmercury was transferred from mother to fetus via the placenta. The developing brain of the fetus was thus heavily exposed to methylmercury. Consequently, fetuses were more severely afflicted with central nervous system disorders, named "congenital *Minamata* disease." The affected fetuses are considered to act as a sink for methylmercury, thus mitigating the severity of toxicity in the mother [14]. However, it should be pointed out that congenital *Minamata* disease does not directly go with the DOHaD theory because newborn babies have manifested devastatingly abnormal signs and symptoms soon after birth without a latency period. In addition, histopathologic examination of brain tissue obtained from patients at necropsy revealed conspicuous degeneration of neuronal tissue. It should be noted that the congenital *Minamata* disease is regarded as the most extreme end of the spectrum of methylmercury poisoning. However, it is conceivable that pregnant women who are exposed to methylmercury at low doses that do not induce conspicuous abnormalities may deliver newborn babies who might develop behavioral or cognitive abnormalities later in life, which may fit into the DOHaD paradigm, as described below. Besides methylmercury poisoning, other chemical poisoning cases, including DES, dioxin/PCBs, and arsenic, may also reflect the extreme end of the spectrum of abnormal phenotypes.

1.4 Prenatal Chemical Exposure and Late-Onset Cancers in Offspring

Prenatal exposure to the pharmaceutical diethylstilbestrol (DES) is considered to be adopted as a proof of principle to study the DOHaD paradigm [15]. DES is a potent synthetic estrogen and was extensively prescribed in the USA, Canada, and some European countries to pregnant women from the 1940s to the 1970s. In these countries, this drug was mistakenly believed to prevent miscarriage, premature labor, and related complications of pregnancy [16]. It is estimated that over ten million people were exposed only in the USA and that 1/1000 developed cancer of the cervix and vagina in offspring who were born to DES-prescribed mothers during pregnancy. Furthermore, other health problems including a higher incidence of breast cancer in women and testicular abnormalities (undescended testicles and epididymal cysts) in men born to mothers who were treated with DES have been noted. However, the association is not clear-cut, and definitive conclusions cannot be drawn [16, 17].

As to the possible occurrence of DES-related health problems in Japan, no English language papers that report the prescription of DES to pregnant women in Japan are available. Mizutani intensively examined Japanese literature that reported the DES situation in Japan and published a book on DES poisoning [18]. Since this is the only book so far published on the DES situation in Japan, I briefly present his findings, although this topic may not be in the mainstream of this review. First, in Japan, DES and its derivatives were introduced to the market between 1940 and 1960 but banned for use in pregnant women by the Ministry of Health in December, 1971. Second, the dose of DES contained in a pellet sold in Japan was approximately 1 mg/day, which was much lower than the dose recommended for use in the USA (5–125 mg/day). Third, literature analysis indicated that hormone treatment for premature delivery or miscarriage using DES and its derivatives adopted in the USA and other countries did not receive strong support from Japanese obstetricians/gynecologists after its introduction in Japan but instead received criticism. Overall, Mizutani [18] concluded that DES treatment was introduced to obstetrics and gynecology practice in Japan on a very limited scale and did not become common practice.

The late-onset abnormalities observed in the offspring born to mothers administered DES during gestation have been supported by many experimental studies. McLachlan and colleagues [19] showed that male mice offspring (60%) born to dams exposed to DES were sterile with intra-abdominal or fibrotic testes or both and that nodular masses were observed in the ampullary region of the reproductive tract in 6 of 24 animals, with 1 undergoing a seemingly preneoplastic change. Nomura and associates [20] reported that DES was transferred to the fetus via placenta and that a critical window exists during gestation (days 15–19). They found that female offspring was sensitive to abnormalities in the uterus and vagina and that male offspring was susceptible to have undescended testes and hypogenesis. They also found that the incidence of various tumors (lung adenoma, granulosa cell tumor, etc.) increased significantly when DES was given in the critical window (days 15 and 17), which correspond to the stage that is sensitive to other carcinogens. However, adenosis and adenocarcinoma of the vagina were not observed in the offspring. These animal models as well as other later studies strongly support the mechanism of DES toxicity in human cases.

It is well-known that a prolonged latency period, often up to several years, is required for the pathogenesis of cancers, regardless of the cause. Yamagiwa and Ichikawa first established a chemical carcinogenesis animal model in 1915, by topically applying coal tar for hundreds of days to produce carcinoma in the rabbit ear [21]. A representative chemical carcinogenesis model has been established as two-stage or multistage model. The stages comprise of initiation, promotion, and progression [22]. The DES-induced cancers may fit into a model of a chemical carcinogenesis. However, DES-induced cancers have features distinct from the chemically induced skin or colon cancers; the former has a very narrow critical window in the neonatal period [23], whereas the latter does not and occurs during adulthood.

1.5 Prenatal Chemical Exposure and Neurobehavioral and Cognitive Abnormalities

Epidemiologic and animal studies have shown that the developing brain is extremely vulnerable to exogenous chemicals (Fig. 1.1). Although at least 80,000 synthetic chemicals have been on the market, many potential neurotoxicants have not been identified or examined for developmental neurotoxicity because of the costs involved or absence of a legal requirement [24]. It should be pointed out that in the Heindel review [13], tobacco- and alcohol-related papers were not included; had they been included as keywords, the number of papers may have increased. Grandjean and Landrigan [25] reported that at least a dozen exogenous chemicals act as neurotoxicants, which include lead, methylmercury, polychlorinated biphenyls, arsenic, toluene, manganese, fluoride, chlorpyrifos, dichlorodiphenyltrichloroethane, tetrachloroethylene, and polybrominated diphenyl ethers. From risk assessment based on environmental health point of view, we need to consider that late-onset abnormalities may be caused by prenatal exposure to low-dose chemicals that do not overly harm pregnant women as well as their fetuses. Moreover, subtle alterations not detected by routine diagnostic procedures, presumably induced by epigenetic mechanisms, may also cause such abnormalities. Such exposure scenarios may fall into the DOHaD paradigm.

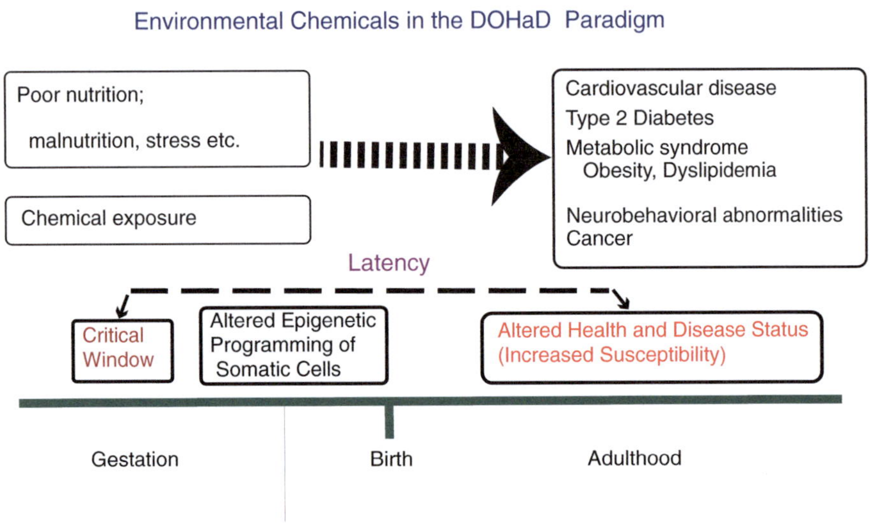

Fig. 1.1 A scheme of the DOHaD paradigm with regard to chemical exposure

Majority of the neurotoxicants have physicochemical properties like low molecular weight and high lipophilicity that help them penetrate the fetoplacental and blood-brain barriers and may elicit toxicity because these barriers normally block the entry of chemicals into the brain parenchyma. Exposure assessment data show that environmental levels of these chemicals are frequently detected in food material. Thus, it is conceivable that they are ingested by pregnant women through food and transferred to the fetus, leading to adverse effects on growth and development of fetal tissue and eventually inducing late-onset abnormalities in their developing brain. If prenatal rather than postnatal exposure is more likely to lead to adverse health outcomes, the etiology can be considered to fall in into the spectrum of DOHaD.

The following are some examples of the chemicals that induce developmental neurotoxicity that fits into the DOHaD concept.

Methylmercury. The primary source of methylmercury exposure in daily life is consumption of higher trophic level fish, like bluefin tuna and swordfish, and marine mammals, like whales and dolphins. No conspicuous abnormalities are diagnosed by physicians with daily exposure to environmental levels of methylmercury, which is in contrast to the severe symptoms of *Minamata* disease or Iraqi poisoning victims. However, subtle neurodevelopmental effects have been observed in populations with moderate methylmercury exposures in a cohort study in the Faeroe Islands where whales have been traditionally caught and consumed for a living. For example, in a study on 878 offspring, who were 14 years old, indicators of prenatal methylmercury exposure were significantly associated with deficits in finger tapping speed, reaction time on a continued performance task, and cued naming. In the islands belonging to the Republic of Seychelles, a target population of pairs of mothers and infants who were exposed to methylmercury mainly via various kinds of fish were subjected to a cohort study. Results from the Seychelles cohort studies were used to derive NOAEL of methylmercury in infants. These epidemiological study results were used to derive provisional tolerable intake level by the Joint FAO/WHO Expert Committee on Food Additives (JECFA) [26].

Arsenic. Over 20 million people are exposed to arsenic-contaminated water worldwide, such as Bangladesh, China, India, Chile, and many other countries. The WHO's current recommended limit of arsenic in drinking water is 10 μg/L, although this level is designated as provisional because of measurement difficulties and the practical difficulties in removing arsenic from drinking water [27]. In the city of Antofagasta in northern Chile, more than 250,000 people were exposed to a high arsenic content in drinking water (870 μg/L) from 1958 until 1970 when exposure was terminated by installation and operation of an arsenic removal plant. The epidemiologic studies carried out in this area have some advantages over similar studies in other parts of the world for clarifying dose-response relationship. The lifetime exposure and long-term latency patterns can be assessed with better accuracy from the Antofagasta studies because of its unique geology, limited water sources, and good historical records [28]. Evidence of increased mortality from lung cancer, bronchiectasis, myocardial infarction, and kidney cancer has been reported among young adults who were born when tap water was highly contaminated with arsenic between 1958 and 1970 or were less than 18 years old. In addition, epidemiologic studies carried out between 2007 and 2010, approximately 40 years after the cessation of high-level arsenic exposure, indicate a high prevalence of lung and bladder cancer. It is concluded that exposure to arsenic in utero or during infancy may enhance the tendency to getting afflicted with the abovementioned diseases [29]. These observations are important in terms of risk assessment of arsenic because some food commodities contained non-negligible concentrations of inorganic arsenic, including *hijiki*, a kind of seaweed. An alert not to eat this seaweed has been issued in the UK, whereas *hijiki* is commonly consumed by the Japanese population.

Tobacco. Smoking during pregnancy predisposes the fetus to many kinds of potentially hazardous chemicals. Nicotine and carbon monoxide are typical chemicals, both of which penetrate the fetoplacental barrier. Adverse effects of prenatal smoking exposure have been well-documented. Growth of the body and the head of the fetus can be hampered, and alterations in brain structure and function can be seen in children who are exposed to prenatal smoking. In addition to these short-term effects, prenatal smoking was found to alter cardiovascular function (blood pressure control and heart rate response) 1 year after birth [30]. Altered function of the nicotinic acetylcholine receptor (nAChR) by prenatal nicotine exposure is closely involved in the abnormal development of the brain. Nicotine exposure during pregnancy has been shown to affect brain cell replication and differentiation, leading to changes in brain structure, such as impaired growth of the rat forebrain [31]. Tobacco smoking during pregnancy also elevates carbon monoxide concentration not only in maternal blood but also in fetal blood because it can pass through the placenta. Carbon monoxide binds to hemoglobin and produces carboxyhemoglobin, which impairs oxygen delivery to the fetus. Furthermore, prenatal nicotine exposure was found to affect the contractility of the uterine arteries and to decrease uterine blood flow in pregnant animals [32]. Therefore, maternal smoking during pregnancy can lead to fetal hypoxia and ischemia, which may disrupt normal growth and development of the fetal brain.

Prenatal passive smoking was inversely associated with neurodevelopmental outcomes in young children, whereas postnatal passive smoking was associated with poor academic achievement and neurocognitive performance in older children and adolescents. Furthermore, Chen and associates [33] systematically reviewed articles (dated 1989–2012) that investigated the association between passive smoking, focusing on prenatal exposure by pregnant women, and performance on neurocognitive and academic tests. It was confirmed that passive smoking by pregnant women showed a strong association with reduced neurodevelopment especially in children aged younger than 5 years, even after controlling for postnatal passive smoking. Children, on an individual basis, who were prenatally exposed to passive smoking were in a normal range in cognitive performance, but on a group basis, their cognitive performance was lower than those who were not exposed. The literature on passive smoking during prenatal and postnatal periods consistently indicates associations with increased rates of behavior problems, including irritability, oppositional defiant behavior, conduct disorders, and attention deficit hyperactivity disorder, although the relative roles of prenatal vs. postnatal exposure have not been studied [34].

Humans are exposed to pesticides through food and environment. Because of the accumulated knowledge on health problems in children from daily exposure to pesticides, the American Academy of Pediatrics [35] published a position paper, stating that epidemiologic evidence demonstrates associations between early life exposure to pesticides and pediatric cancers, decreased cognitive function, and behavioral problems. Biomonitoring of urinary organophosphate metabolites indicated associations of exposure to organophosphates with neurotoxicity outcomes, including poor mental development, attention-deficit/hyperactivity disorder, low IQ scores, and parent-reported behavioral problems [36–41].

Among OP pesticides, chlorpyrifos (CPF) has been widely used as a broad-spectrum organophosphate insecticide for pest control. Prenatal exposure to CPF is associated with neurobehavioral deficits in humans and animal models. Rauh and associates [39] investigated the association between CPF exposure and brain morphology using magnetic resonance imaging in 40 children (5.9–11.2 years old), selected from a nonclinical, representative community-based cohort. When the subjects were categorized by CPF concentrations in umbilical cord blood, a significant association was observed between prenatal exposure to CPF and structural changes in the developing human brain. Although the route of exposure to pesticides can be multiple, an intervention study clearly demonstrated that the most influential route of exposure is through the diet. In that study, diet was replaced with organic food items for 5 consecutive days, and urine specimens were collected from 23 children for 2 weeks including the intervention period. Urinary levels of organophosphates pesticides showed that metabolites for malathion and chlorpyrifos decreased to the undetectable levels immediately after the introduction of organic diet and remained so until conventional diet was reintroduced [42].

Recently, organophosphorus pesticides have been gradually replaced with neonicotinoid pesticides, and the total amounts of production of OPs decreased from approximately 6000 tons in 2000 to approximately 2000 tons in 2011. The use of neonicotinoid pesticides for pest control has been registered in more than 120 countries in the world, with global production being valued at US$2.5 billion [43]. According to a recent study on exposure assessment of OPs and neonicotinoids [44], urine specimens obtained from Japanese women during the period 1994–2011 indicate a decreasing trend of the excreted amounts of OPs and an increasing trend of neonicotinoids (acetamiprid, clothianidin, dinotefuran, imidacloprid, nitenpyram, thiacloprid, and thiamethoxam). More importantly, it should be borne in mind that neonicotinoids, as well as organophosphates and pyrethroids, that were not naturally present in humans were detected in urine specimens from infants ([45]; Ikenaka et al., personal communication). Sano et al. [46] reported that only male mice born to dams administered with acetamiprid from gestational day 6 to lactation day 21 showed abnormalities in sociosexual and anxiety-related behaviors, without a change in the testosterone level. An excitatory action of acetamiprid or imidacloprid on neurons via nicotinic acetylcholine receptor subtypes was shown by an in vitro study using primary cultures of cerebellar neurons from neonatal rats [47]. Thus, it is reasonable to consider that OPs, neonicotinoids, and possibly PYRs in food commodities are absorbed by pregnant women and infants and retained for a prolonged time to induce abnormalities in the developing brain and lead to other disease states.

Dioxins. Polychlorinated dibenzo-*p*-dioxin (PCDD), dibenzofuran (PCDF), and biphenyl (PCB) congeners are persistent, and ubiquitous environmental contaminants that are found in air, water, soil, and sediment bioaccumulate in various animal species including humans worldwide. PCDDs and PCDFs are unintentional byproducts of combustion and various industrial activities. PCB mixtures were commercial products widely used as heat-resistant solvents and lubricants and in fluorescent light ballasts before they were banned. A subset of PCDD, PCDF, and PCB congeners can bind and activate aryl hydrocarbon receptor (AhR) to exert various kinds of toxicities, such as metabolic disorders, reproductive toxicity and neurodevelopmental toxicity, immunosuppression, and carcinogenicity, and referred as dioxin-like (DL) congeners or simply as dioxins [48]. Among them, 2,3,7,8-tetrachlorodibenzo-*p*-dioxin (TCDD) is the most potent in causing toxicity and is the prototype to which biological and toxicological actions of all other DL-congeners are compared. With regard to the DOHaD paradigm, it is important to point out that in utero and lactational exposure to low dose of TCDD was shown to induce toxicity phenotypes in rodents and nonhuman primates, such as abnormalities in higher brain function, sexual differentiation (demasculinization), and immune dysfunction, in offspring during adulthood. It has been established that AhR is essential for the manifestation of the majority of toxicity phenotypes, but the morphological and functional cause that determines toxicity phenotypes beyond AhR signaling remains largely unstudied [49].

1.6 Alterations During Gestation That May Link Chemical Exposure and the DOHaD Phenotypes

Pathogenesis of lifestyle-related diseases that the DOHaD paradigm relies on differs by disease phenotypes, although the commonality of the pathogenesis is that a factor(s) during the gestational and neonatal periods could affect the health status of the offspring. In the case of chemical exposure, perinatal exposure to low-dose chemical exposure has been known to affect function of the developing brain, which results in abnormalities in cognitive and behavioral functions later in adulthood. However, the underlying mechanisms that link chemical exposure and the health outcomes are largely unknown.

A battery of behavioral tests as well as histopathologic techniques recommended for use in developmental toxicity testing by OECD test guideline 426 may lack reliability and detection sensitivity [24]. For example, the number of pesticides that were said to be subjected to these DNT test guidelines is extremely limited, and almost no endpoints have been used to derive allowable daily intake (ADI) [24]. In other words, in order to minimize the potential for developmental neurotoxicity, the application of cutting-edge techniques to the hypothesis-driven DNT testing is likely to be able to detect subtle or early-phase alteratons in the offspring [50].

A given chemical, which belongs to a group of EDCs and has an estrogenic or androgenic activity, may induce neurobehavioral disturbances by disrupting sex hormone receptor-mediated mechanisms. Mammalian brain is sexually differentiated during perinatal period by estradiol, which is aromatized in the brain from androgen synthesized in the fetal and neonatal testis. Female brains were protected by plasma glycoproteins that bind circulating estrogens. The amount of steroid in well-established sexually dimorphic regions is typically higher than that in the hippocampus and cortex and may be due to a combination of regionally specific uptake, synthesis, and metabolism [51]. Thus, it is reasonable to suspect that bisphenol A (BPA) may have such an effect.

Bisphenol A has been widely used in the production of polycarbonate plastics, epoxy resins used to line metal cans, and numerous plastic consumer products and has been most extensively studied and evaluated for endocrine-disrupting activities with regard to risk assessment purposes [52]. Perinatal exposure to low doses of BPA downregulated the expression levels of estrogen receptor α and β in sexual dimorphic regions, anteroventral periventricular nucleus (AVPV), and medial preoptic area (MPOA) in the hypothalamus of rats. BPA has been known to interact with ERα and ERβ and has been shown to interfere with hippocampal synaptogenesis [53, 54].

An application of cutting-edge techniques, which are not meant to be used in the toxicology test guidelines, revealed that perinatal exposure of BPA, TCDD, or other chemicals may induce abnormalities at the neuronal micromorphology level in brain regions, such as hippocampus and amygdala that govern learning/memory and memory, respectively. Perinatal BPA exposure to rodents was found to induce morphological abnormalities in neuronal development [55]. Prenatal exposure to a low-dose BPA

(40 or 400 μg/kg body weight per day) impaired not only the branching of dendrites of hippocampal neurons at an earlier developmental stage but also dendritic spine density in a hippocampal subregion during adulthood. It is shown that such alterations that occurred during brain development persist to adulthood and lead to behavioral and cognitive abnormalities, such as anxiety-like behavior, loss of exploration, learning/ and memory, socio-sexual behaviors across mammalian species [56–59], and social recognition difficulties [60]. However, the molecular basis of such behavioral and cognitive disorders is not fully understood. No study has conclusively shown that BPA altered Dnmt expression or chromatin modification after BPA exposure influences sexual differentiation of the brain in adulthood [61].

Rodent offspring born to dams administered with a low-dose TCDD has been shown to manifest cognitive and behavioral abnormalities, such as spatial, reversal, and alternate and paired associate learning and memory, as well as anxiety and sociality in adulthood [62–69]. In mice offspring under the identical TCDD exposure conditions as in our laboratory, 14-day-old mice exhibited disrupted dendritic branch growth in both the hippocampus and amygdala, and 16-month-old mice had significantly reduced spine densities in the hippocampus [70]. Prenatal exposure to TCDD was found to disrupt the gene expression of glutamate receptor subunits and BDNF, the molecules that control spatial learning and epigenetic-mediated learning, respectively, in the hippocampus and cerebral cortex [71, 72] and induced imbalance of neural activity between the prefrontal cortex and amygdala [62].

Taken together, it is concluded that the micromorphological evidence on BPA- or TCDD-exposed developing brain links chemical exposure with cognitive and behavioral abnormalities. It is implicated that scrutiny using the most appropriate and sensitive state-of-the-art assays [50] that can determine minute alterations, such as neuronal morphology, is needed in developmental neurotoxicity testing in order to clarify the underlying mechanisms of the DOHaD paradigm.

1.7 Conclusion

The DOHaD paradigm has been gaining increasing interest from various disciplines of medical science. Researches on the prenatal low-dose exposure to environmental and industrial chemicals, such as heavy metals, pesticides, tobacco, alcohol, dioxins, and diethylstilbestrol, have revealed that not only the poor nutritional status during gestation but also prenatal chemical exposure may have some characteristics, such as critical window and latency between the time of exposure and health outcomes, in common with the DOHaD paradigm. The nature of the mechanisms underlying the abnormal health outcomes induced by chemical exposure with regard to the DOHaD paradigm is largely unknown. In particular, to clarify the underlying mechanisms of developmental neurotoxicity in the context of the DOHaD paradigm, the most appropriate and sensitive state-of-the-art assays that can detect subtle changes at the micromorphological or molecular levels based on a hypothesis-driven approach are needed.

References

1. Inadera H. Developmental origins of obesity and type 2 diabetes: molecular aspects and role of chemicals. Environ Health Prev Med. 2013;18(3):185–97. https://doi.org/10.1007/s12199-013-0328-8.
2. Gluckman PD, Hanson MA, Cooper C, Thornburg KL. Effect of in utero and early-life conditions on adult health and disease. N Engl J Med. 2008;359(1):61–73. https://doi.org/10.1056/NEJMra0708473.
3. Godfrey KM, Barker DJ. Fetal programming and adult health. Public Health Nutr. 2001;4(2B):611–24.
4. Gillman MW, Barker D, Bier D, Cagampang F, Challis J, Fall C, et al. Meeting report on the 3rd International Congress on Developmental Origins of Health and Disease (DOHaD). Pediatr Res. 2007;61(5 Pt 1):625–9. https://doi.org/10.1203/pdr.0b013e3180459fcd.
5. Colborn T. Pesticides—how research has succeeded and failed to translate science into policy: endocrinological effects on wildlife. Environ Health Perspect. 1995;103(Suppl 6):81–5.
6. Colborn T, Dumanoski D, Myers JP. Our stolen future: are we threatening our fertility, intelligence, and survival?—a scientific detective story. New York: The Spieler Agency; 1996.
7. International Programme on Chemical Safety. Global assessment of the state-of-the-science of endocrine disruptors. Geneva: World Health Organisation; 2002.
8. Barker DJ, Eriksson JG, Forsen T, Osmond C. Infant growth and income 50 years later. Arch Dis Child. 2005;90(3):272–3. https://doi.org/10.1136/adc.2003.033464.
9. Grun F, Blumberg B. Perturbed nuclear receptor signaling by environmental obesogens as emerging factors in the obesity crisis. Rev Endocr Metab Disord. 2007;8(2):161–71. https://doi.org/10.1007/s11154-007-9049-x.
10. Bezek S, Ujhazy E, Mach M, Navarova J, Dubovicky M. Developmental origin of chronic diseases: toxicological implication. Interdiscip Toxicol. 2008;1(1):29–31. https://doi.org/10.2478/v10102-010-0029-8.
11. Grandjean P, Bellinger D, Bergman A, Cordier S, Davey-Smith G, Eskenazi B, et al. The faroes statement: human health effects of developmental exposure to chemicals in our environment. Basic Clin Pharmacol Toxicol. 2008;102(2):73–5. https://doi.org/10.1111/j.1742-7843.2007.00114.x.
12. Rosenfeld CS. Effects of maternal diet and exposure to bisphenol A on sexually dimorphic responses in conceptuses and offspring. Reprod Domest Anim. 2012;47(Suppl 4):23–30. https://doi.org/10.1111/j.1439-0531.2012.02051.x.
13. Heindel JJ, Skalla LA, Joubert BR, Dilworth CH, Gray KA. Review of developmental origins of health and disease publications in environmental epidemiology. Reprod Toxicol. 2017;68:34–48. https://doi.org/10.1016/j.reprotox.2016.11.011.
14. Harada M. Minamata disease: methylmercury poisoning in Japan caused by environmental pollution. Crit Rev Toxicol. 1995;25(1):1–24. https://doi.org/10.3109/10408449509089885.
15. Newbold RR. Prenatal exposure to diethylstilbestrol and long-term impact on the breast and reproductive tract in humans and mice. J Dev Orig Health Dis. 2012;3(2):73–82. https://doi.org/10.1017/S2040174411000754.
16. National Cancer Institute. Diethylstilbestrol (DES) and Cancer. https://www.cancer.gov/about-cancer/causes-prevention/risk/hormones/des-fact-sheet.
17. Larson PS, Ungarelli RA, de Las Morenas A, Cupples LA, Rowlings K, Palmer JR, et al. In utero exposure to diethylstilbestrol (DES) does not increase genomic instability in normal or neoplastic breast epithelium. Cancer. 2006;107(9):2122–6. https://doi.org/10.1002/cncr.22223.
18. Mizutani T. DES Yakugai. Tokyo: Hon-no-izumi Co.; 2004.
19. McLachlan JA, Newbold RR, Bullock B. Reproductive tract lesions in male mice exposed prenatally to diethylstilbestrol. Science. 1975;190(4218):991–2.
20. Nomura T, Kanzaki T. Induction of urogenital anomalies and some tumors in the progeny of mice receiving diethylstilbestrol during pregnancy. Cancer Res. 1977;37(4):1099–104.

21. Weisburger JH. Nakahara memorial lecture. Application of the mechanisms of nutritional carcinogenesis to the prevention of cancer. Princess Takamatsu Symp. 1985;16:11–26.
22. Abel EL, Angel JM, Kiguchi K, DiGiovanni J. Multi-stage chemical carcinogenesis in mouse skin: fundamentals and applications. Nat Protoc. 2009;4(9):1350–62. https://doi.org/10.1038/nprot.2009.120.
23. Newbold RR, McLachlan JA. Vaginal adenosis and adenocarcinoma in mice exposed prenatally or neonatally to diethylstilbestrol. Cancer Res. 1982;42(5):2003–11.
24. Tohyama C. Developmental neurotoxicity guidelines: problems and perspectives. J Toxicol Sci. 2016;41(Special):SP69–79. https://doi.org/10.2131/jts.41.SP69.
25. Grandjean P, Landrigan PJ. Neurobehavioural effects of developmental toxicity. Lancet Neurol. 2014;13(3):330–8. https://doi.org/10.1016/S1474-4422(13)70278-3.
26. WHO. Evaluation of certain food additives and contaminants. Sixty-first report of the Joint FAO/WHO Expert Committee on Food Additives. Geneva: WHO; 2004.
27. WHO. Arsenic fact sheet. 2016. http://www.who.int/mediacentre/factsheets/fs372/en/.
28. Smith AH, Marshall G, Liaw J, Yuan Y, Ferreccio C, Steinmaus C. Mortality in young adults following in utero and childhood exposure to arsenic in drinking water. Environ Health Perspect. 2012;120(11):1527–31. https://doi.org/10.1289/ehp.1104867.
29. Steinmaus CM, Ferreccio C, Romo JA, Yuan Y, Cortes S, Marshall G, et al. Drinking water arsenic in northern Chile: high cancer risks 40 years after exposure cessation. Cancer Epidemiol Biomark Prev. 2013;22(4):623–30. https://doi.org/10.1158/1055-9965.EPI-12-1190.
30. Cohen G, Jeffery H, Lagercrantz H, Katz-Salamon M. Long-term reprogramming of cardiovascular function in infants of active smokers. Hypertension. 2010;55(3):722–8. https://doi.org/10.1161/HYPERTENSIONAHA.109.142695.
31. Ekblad M, Korkeila J, Lehtonen L. Smoking during pregnancy affects foetal brain development. Acta Paediatr. 2015;104(1):12–8. https://doi.org/10.1111/apa.12791.
32. Xiao D, Huang X, Yang S, Zhang L. Direct effects of nicotine on contractility of the uterine artery in pregnancy. J Pharmacol Exp Ther. 2007;322(1):180–5. https://doi.org/10.1124/jpet.107.119354.
33. Chen R, Clifford A, Lang L, Anstey KJ. Is exposure to secondhand smoke associated with cognitive parameters of children and adolescents?—a systematic literature review. Ann Epidemiol. 2013;23(10):652–61. https://doi.org/10.1016/j.annepidem.2013.07.001.
34. Herrmann M, King K, Weitzman M. Prenatal tobacco smoke and postnatal secondhand smoke exposure and child neurodevelopment. Curr Opin Pediatr. 2008;20(2):184–90. https://doi.org/10.1097/MOP.0b013e3282f56165.
35. Council on Environmental Health. Pesticide exposure in children. Pediatrics. 2012;130(6):e1757–63. https://doi.org/10.1542/peds.2012-2757.
36. Bouchard MF, Bellinger DC, Wright RO, Weisskopf MG. Attention-deficit/hyperactivity disorder and urinary metabolites of organophosphate pesticides. Pediatrics. 2010;125(6):e1270–7. https://doi.org/10.1542/peds.2009-3058.
37. Bouchard MF, Chevrier J, Harley KG, Kogut K, Vedar M, Calderon N, et al. Prenatal exposure to organophosphate pesticides and IQ in 7-year-old children. Environ Health Perspect. 2011;119(8):1189–95. https://doi.org/10.1289/ehp.1003185.
38. Rauh V, Arunajadai S, Horton M, Perera F, Hoepner L, Barr DB, et al. Seven-year neurodevelopmental scores and prenatal exposure to chlorpyrifos, a common agricultural pesticide. Environ Health Perspect. 2011;119(8):1196–201. https://doi.org/10.1289/ehp.1003160.
39. Rauh VA, Perera FP, Horton MK, Whyatt RM, Bansal R, Hao X, et al. Brain anomalies in children exposed prenatally to a common organophosphate pesticide. Proc Natl Acad Sci U S A. 2012;109(20):7871–6. https://doi.org/10.1073/pnas.1203396109.
40. Sanchez-Santed F, Colomina MT, Herrero Hernandez E. Organophosphate pesticide exposure and neurodegeneration. Cortex. 2016;74:417–26. https://doi.org/10.1016/j.cortex.2015.10.003.
41. Stallones L, Beseler CL. Assessing the connection between organophosphate pesticide poisoning and mental health: a comparison of neuropsychological symptoms from clinical observations, animal models and epidemiological studies. Cortex. 2016;74:405–16. https://doi.org/10.1016/j.cortex.2015.10.002.

42. Lu C, Toepel K, Irish R, Fenske RA, Barr DB, Bravo R. Organic diets significantly lower children's dietary exposure to organophosphorus pesticides. Environ Health Perspect. 2006;114(2):260–3.
43. Sadaria AM, Supowit SD, Halden RU. Halden mass balance assessment for six neonicotinoid insecticides during conventional wastewater and wetland treatment: nationwide reconnaissance in United States wastewater. Environ Sci Technol. 2016;50:6199–206. https://doi.org/10.1021/acs.est.6b01032.
44. Ueyama J, Harada KH, Koizumi A, Sugiura Y, Kondo T, Saito I, et al. Temporal levels of urinary neonicotinoid and dialkylphosphate concentrations in Japanese women between 1994 and 2011. Environ Sci Technol. 2015;49(24):14522–8. https://doi.org/10.1021/acs.est.5b03062.
45. Osaka A, Ueyama J, Kondo T, Nomura H, Sugiura Y, Saito I, et al. Exposure characterization of three major insecticide lines in urine of young children in Japan-neonicotinoids, organophosphates, and pyrethroids. Environ Res. 2016;147:89–96. https://doi.org/10.1016/j.envres.2016.01.028.
46. Sano K, Isobe T, Yang J, Win-Shwe TT, Yoshikane M, Nakayama SF, et al. In utero and lactational exposure to acetamiprid induces abnormalities in socio-sexual and anxiety-related behaviors of male mice. Front Neurosci. 2016;10:228. https://doi.org/10.3389/fnins.2016.00228.
47. Kimura-Kuroda J, Komuta Y, Kuroda Y, Hayashi M, Kawano H. Nicotine-like effects of the neonicotinoid insecticides acetamiprid and imidacloprid on cerebellar neurons from neonatal rats. PLoS One. 2012;7(2):e32432. https://doi.org/10.1371/journal.pone.0032432.
48. Schecter A, Gasiewicz TA, editors. Dioxin and health. 2nd ed. Hoboken: Wiley; 2005. https://doi.org/10.1002/0471722014.
49. Yoshioka W, Peterson RE, Tohyama C. Molecular targets that link dioxin exposure to toxicity phenotypes. J Steroid Biochem Mol Biol. 2011;127(1–2):96–101. https://doi.org/10.1016/j.jsbmb.2010.12.005.
50. Myers JP, vom Saal FS, Akingbemi BT, Arizono K, Belcher S, Colborn T, et al. Why public health agencies cannot depend on good laboratory practices as a criterion for selecting data: the case of bisphenol A. Environ Health Perspect. 2009;117(3):309–15. https://doi.org/10.1289/ehp.0800173.
51. Konkle AT, McCarthy MM. Developmental time course of estradiol, testosterone, and dihydrotestosterone levels in discrete regions of male and female rat brain. Endocrinology. 2011;152(1):223–35. https://doi.org/10.1210/en.2010-0607.
52. EFSA Panel on Food Contact Materials, Enzymes, Flavourings and Processing Aids. Scientific Opinion on the risks to public health related to the presence of bisphenol A (BPA) in foodstuffs: executive summary. 2015. https://efsa.onlinelibrary.wiley.com/doi/abs/10.2903/j.efsa.2015.3978. Accessed 20 Sept 2018.
53. Leranth C, Hajszan T, Szigeti-Buck K, Bober J, MacLusky NJ. Bisphenol A prevents the synaptogenic response to estradiol in hippocampus and prefrontal cortex of ovariectomized nonhuman primates. Proc Natl Acad Sci U S A. 2008;105(37):14187–91. https://doi.org/10.1073/pnas.0806139105.
54. MacLusky NJ, Hajszan T, Leranth C. The environmental estrogen bisphenol A inhibits estradiol-induced hippocampal synaptogenesis. Environ Health Perspect. 2005;113(6):675–9.
55. Kimura E, Matsuyoshi C, Miyazaki W, Benner S, Hosokawa M, Yokoyama K, et al. Prenatal exposure to bisphenol A impacts neuronal morphology in the hippocampal CA1 region in developing and aged mice. Arch Toxicol. 2016;90(3):691–700. https://doi.org/10.1007/s00204-015-1485-x.
56. Poimenova A, Markaki E, Rahiotis C, Kitraki E. Corticosterone-regulated actions in the rat brain are affected by perinatal exposure to low dose of bisphenol A. Neuroscience. 2010;167(3):741–9. https://doi.org/10.1016/j.neuroscience.2010.02.051.
57. Tian YH, Baek JH, Lee SY, Jang CG. Prenatal and postnatal exposure to bisphenol a induces anxiolytic behaviors and cognitive deficits in mice. Synapse. 2010;64(6):432–9. https://doi.org/10.1002/syn.20746.
58. Xu X, Hong X, Xie L, Li T, Yang Y, Zhang Q, et al. Gestational and lactational exposure to bisphenol-A affects anxiety- and depression-like behaviors in mice. Horm Behav. 2012;62(4):480–90.

59. Luo G, Wang S, Li Z, Wei R, Zhang L, Liu H, et al. Maternal bisphenol a diet induces anxiety-like behavior in female juvenile with neuroimmune activation. Toxicol Sci. 2014;140(2):364–73. https://doi.org/10.1093/toxsci/kfu085.
60. Wolstenholme JT, Goldsby JA, Rissman EF. Transgenerational effects of prenatal bisphenol A on social recognition. Horm Behav. 2013;64(5):833–9. https://doi.org/10.1016/j.yhbeh.2013.09.007.
61. Walker DM, Gore AC. Epigenetic impacts of endocrine disruptors in the brain. Front Neuroendocrinol. 2017;44:1–26. https://doi.org/10.1016/j.yfrne.2016.09.002.
62. Endo T, Kakeyama M, Uemura Y, Haijima A, Okuno H, Bito H, et al. Executive function deficits and social-behavioral abnormality in mice exposed to a low dose of dioxin in utero and via lactation. PLoS One. 2012;7(12):e50741. https://doi.org/10.1371/journal.pone.0050741.
63. Haijima A, Endo T, Zhang Y, Miyazaki W, Kakeyama M, Tohyama C. In utero and lactational exposure to low doses of chlorinated and brominated dioxins induces deficits in the fear memory of male mice. Neurotoxicology. 2010;31(4):385–90. https://doi.org/10.1016/j.neuro.2010.04.004.
64. Hojo R, Stern S, Zareba G, Markowski VP, Cox C, Kost JT, et al. Sexually dimorphic behavioral responses to prenatal dioxin exposure. Environ Health Perspect. 2002;110(3):247–54.
65. Ishihara K, Warita K, Tanida T, Sugawara T, Kitagawa H, Hoshi N. Does paternal exposure to 2,3,7,8-tetrachlorodibenzo-p-dioxin (TCDD) affect the sex ratio of offspring? J Vet Med Sci. 2007;69(4):347–52.
66. Kakeyama M, Endo T, Zhang Y, Miyazaki W, Tohyama C. Disruption of paired-associate learning in rat offspring perinatally exposed to dioxins. Arch Toxicol. 2014;88(3):789–98. https://doi.org/10.1007/s00204-013-1161-y.
67. Markowski VP, Zareba G, Stern S, Cox C, Weiss B. Altered operant responding for motor reinforcement and the determination of benchmark doses following perinatal exposure to low-level 2,3,7,8-tetrachlorodibenzo-p-dioxin. Environ Health Perspect. 2001;109(6):621–7.
68. Mitsui T, Sugiyama N, Maeda S, Tohyama C, Arita J. Perinatal exposure to 2,3,7,8-tetrachlor odibenzo-p-dioxin suppresses contextual fear conditioning-accompanied activation of cyclic AMP response element-binding protein in the hippocampal CA1 region of male rats. Neurosci Lett. 2006;398(3):206–10. https://doi.org/10.1016/j.neulet.2005.12.087.
69. Schantz SL, Seo BW, Moshtaghian J, Peterson RE, Moore RW. Effects of gestational and lactational exposure to TCDD or coplanar PCBs on spatial learning. Neurotoxicol Teratol. 1996;18(3):305–13.
70. Kimura E, Kubo K, Matsuyoshi C, Benner S, Hosokawa M, Endo T, et al. Developmental origin of abnormal dendritic growth in the mouse brain induced by in utero disruption of aryl hydrocarbon receptor signaling. Neurotoxicol Teratol. 2015;52(Pt A):42–50. https://doi.org/10.1016/j.ntt.2015.10.005.
71. Hood DB, Woods L, Brown L, Johnson S, Ebner FF. Gestational 2,3,7,8-tetrachlorodibenzo-p-dioxin exposure effects on sensory cortex function. Neurotoxicology. 2006;27(6):1032–42. https://doi.org/10.1016/j.neuro.2006.05.022.
72. Kakeyama M, Sone H, Miyabara Y, Tohyama C. Perinatal exposure to 2,3,7,8-tetrachlorodi benzo-p-dioxin alters activity-dependent expression of BDNF mRNA in the neocortex and male rat sexual behavior in adulthood. Neurotoxicology. 2003;24(2):207–17. https://doi.org/10.1016/S0161-813X(02)00214-0.

Chapter 2
DOHaD Cohort Studies and Public Health Implications in Japan

Kohta Suzuki

Abstract Because the "Developmental Origins of Health and Disease (DOHaD)" hypothesis recently became widely known in a medical research area, fetal and childhood environment has been drawing more attention. In addition, based on the DOHaD, childhood growth trajectories, which are described by multilevel analysis, might be important in examining the effects of early-life environment. Therefore, it becomes more important to establish epidemiological evidence related to DOHaD from population-based birth cohort studies which include the study that uses the dataset from some public health activities. Moreover, it is also important to apply the findings from these studies to public health. In this chapter, some nationwide and local birth cohort studies and the results related to DOHaD from these studies are introduced. For instance, the association between maternal smoking status during pregnancy and birthweight from "Japanese Environment and Children's Study" which is conducted by the Ministry of Environment, and childhood growth trajectories according to maternal smoking status during pregnancy from Project Koshu, are described.

Keywords Birth cohort study · Public health · Japan

Abbreviations

BMI	Body mass index
CI	Confidence interval
DM	Diabetes mellitus
DOHaD	Developmental Origins of Health and Disease

K. Suzuki
Department of Health and Psychosocial Medicine, Aichi Medical University School of Medicine, Nagakute, Aichi, Japan
e-mail: kohtas@aichi-med-u.ac.jp

F. Sata et al. (eds.), *Pre-emptive Medicine: Public Health Aspects of Developmental Origins of Health and Disease*, Current Topics in Environmental Health and Preventive Medicine, https://doi.org/10.1007/978-981-13-2194-8_2

GDM	Gestational diabetes mellitus
HG	Hyperemesis gravidarum
JECS	Japan Environment and Children's Study
LBW	Low birth weight
NS	Never-smokers
NVP	Nausea and vomiting in early pregnancy
OR	Odds ratio
PIH	Pregnancy-induced hypertension
SD	Standard deviation
SGA	Small-for-gestational-age
SM	Current smokers

2.1 Introduction

In recent years, the "Developmental Origins of Health and Diseases" hypothesis, in addition to the established "fetal programming" and "Barker's hypothesis," has been suggested to clarify the mechanisms of childhood growth and development [1]. These were described as an example of the association between a specific path of growth—consisting of slow growth in fetal life and rapidly increasing body mass index (BMI) as an infant—and the development of adulthood chronic diseases [1–5]. Thus, appropriate fetal growth, a crucial element of these hypotheses, is considered an important factor for the future health of an individual. Some perinatal outcomes, such as low birth weight (LBW) and intrauterine growth restriction, are considered indicators of inappropriate fetal growth. However, descriptions of the study participants from the fetal period are necessary to examine these hypotheses or concepts, and it is difficult to collect information on the fetal period in a timely matter in most birth cohort studies, as participants of these studies are usually recruited after birth, and information on the prenatal period (e.g., maternal lifestyle habits during pregnancy) is collected retrospectively. For instance, in Japan, Ministry of Health, Labour and Welfare is carrying out a nationwide birth cohort study called as "Longitudinal Surveys of Newborns in the twenty-first Century (born in 2001 (the 2001 survey) and 2010 (the 2010 survey))" which are based on birth registration data of vital statistics [6]. These surveys were commenced at birth of participants. Thus, it was impossible to timely obtain the information before birth although the data might be highly representative Japanese population. Therefore, it is necessary to consider some information biases and measurement errors in these studies.

Because it is important to obtain accurate descriptions of maternal and child health status to minimize these biases and errors, recent studies like "Japan Environment and Children's Study (JECS)" have begun during the early pregnancy period [7]. Prior to these recent studies, an ongoing prospective cohort study of pregnant women and their children was initiated in a Japanese rural area called "Project Koshu." Previously, I reported the overview of this study [8]. Although this study has several limitations (e.g., relatively small sample size), some articles have examined the association between fetal environment and childhood growth using the dataset of this study [9–18]. For instance, the relationship between maternal smoking during pregnancy and childhood growth, especially as it pertains to childhood obesity, was examined [9, 11–13].

Because these studies are basically carried out in community settings, it might be relatively easy to apply the results from these studies to public health activities not only in a local area but also a country level. In this chapter, some population-based cohort studies and some findings from these studies which could feedback to the communities are introduced.

2.2 Project Koshu

2.2.1 The Overview of Project Koshu

The Koshu city (formerly Enzan city) administration office and Department of Health Sciences, Interdisciplinary Graduate School, University of Yamanashi cooperatively conduct an ongoing prospective cohort study of pregnant women and their children called Project Koshu, which commenced in 1988. Koshu city is located in the center of Japan. The population of Koshu city is 33,000, with approximately 200 births each year. We expected a high follow-up rate in this project because most of the children do not migrate elsewhere until graduation from junior high schools.

In Japan, pregnant women are encouraged to register their pregnancy at the city office, and their children must be registered. In addition, after birth, children are invited to undergo a medical checkup at ages 1.5, 3, and 5 years. First, to ascertain the lifestyle habits of expectant mothers, we conducted a questionnaire-based survey with expectant mothers who visited the city office to register their pregnancies. Informed consent was obtained prior to the survey. In the study area, over 80% of expectant mothers registered their pregnancy in the first trimester, and almost all registered by 18 gestational weeks. Next, at each medical checkup of the children born to these mothers, we surveyed the lifestyle habits of the children and their mothers by using a questionnaire. Subsequently, at each medical checkup for the children, data on children's growth and physical characteristics were collected, in addition to anthropometric data from elementary and junior high school children, which are measured annually in April, for each grade, according to the Japanese School Health and Safety Law. Therefore, childhood anthropometric data were repeatedly obtained.

Originally, the purpose of this cohort study was to describe current status of maternal and child health in the area. For example, a trend of maternal smoking during pregnancy was previously reported [16]. Then, after accumulating the data from each year, longitudinal datasets were created to examine the association between exposures in fetal and infant periods, such as maternal smoking during pregnancy or childhood sleep duration and childhood growth and development. Thus, depending on the research question, various cohorts could be established. The scheme of Project Koshu is presented in Fig. 2.1.

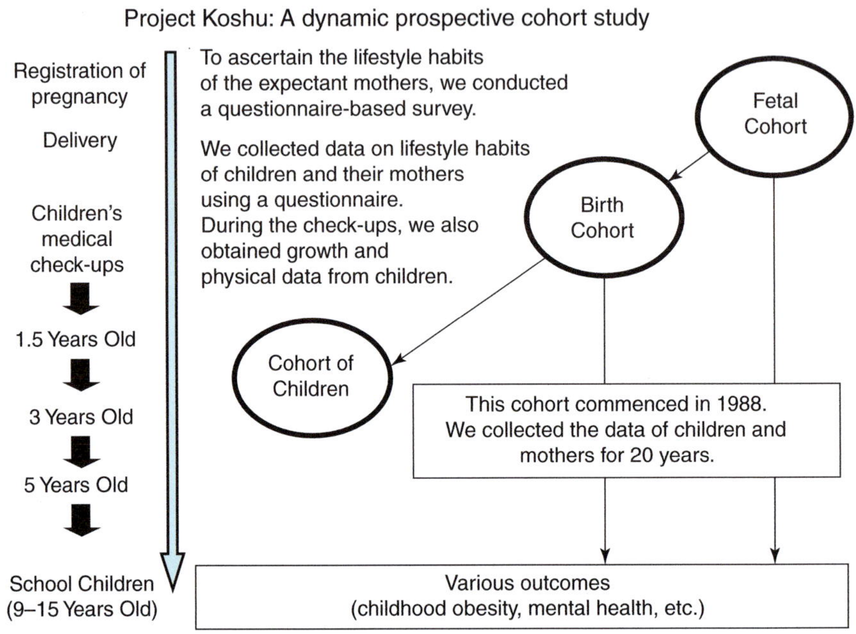

Fig. 2.1 Brief study design of Project Koshu (original data: Suzuki, 2015 [8])

In order to ensure confidentiality, the mothers and children were identified by unique numbers to match the data obtained from the early pregnancy survey and the later medical checkups. This cohort study was approved by the Ethical Review Board of the University of Yamanashi, School of Medicine, and was conducted in accordance with the Guidelines Concerning Epidemiological Research (the Ministry of Education, Culture, Sports, Science, and Technology and the Ministry of Health, Labour and Welfare, Japan). Written informed consent from the participants was obtained.

2.2.2 Some Findings Related to DOHaD from Project Koshu

Maternal smoking during pregnancy is a major cause of low birth weight and intrauterine growth restriction [19–22]. This association has been confirmed in this area [9]. In addition, it has been suggested that maternal smoking cessation before or during early pregnancy may still allow for appropriate fetal and childhood growth [15]. In addition, Mizutani et al. examined the association between maternal lifestyle factors, including smoking during pregnancy, skipping breakfast and short sleep duration, and childhood obesity [9]. This may have been the first article to examine the effect of maternal smoking on childhood obesity in Japan. Maternal smoking habits were significantly associated with overweight (adjusted odds ratio

(OR), 2.2; 95% confidence interval (CI), 1.1–4.1) and obesity (adjusted OR, 3.9; 95% CI, 1.5–10.6) among 5-year-old children [9]. Then, my colleagues and I examined whether the association persists up to 9–10 years of age [11]. However, these point estimates at the age of 9–10 years were considerably lower than those observed at 5 years [11].

Next, we examined the association between maternal smoking during pregnancy and overweight in childhood during different periods using two cohorts from the same population: birth cohort (the first cohort) and non-overweight children at 5 years of age (the second cohort) because there were some differences in adjusted ORs for maternal smoking during pregnancy, which affected the differences observed in childhood obesity/overweight between 5-year-old and 9–10-year-old children [14]. An association between maternal smoking during pregnancy and overweight only in male children in the first cohort analysis (adjusted OR, 4.5; 95% CI, 2.0–10.2) was observed. It is suggested that the effects of maternal smoking during pregnancy on childhood overweight tend to appear before 5 years of age, especially in male children [14].

On the other hand, the term "life course epidemiology" has recently become popular. As previously described, Barker's hypothesis and the DOHaD hypothesis are probably the best-known examples of a life course association. Because these state that poor fetal nutrition, indicated by small birth size, leads to fetal adaptations that alter the propensity to adult diseases [23], it is necessary to describe the growth trajectories during childhood. However, there was no study to carry out such an analysis to clarify the association between maternal lifestyle during pregnancy, which is used as a proxy indicator of fetal environment, and childhood growth or development. Twisk stated that multilevel analysis is usually suitable for analyzing correlated data [24]. Then, my colleagues and I examined the gender differences in the association between maternal smoking during pregnancy and later growth in childhood by conducting a multilevel analysis (a fixed effects model) [12]. The mean birth weight of children whose mothers had smoked during pregnancy was significantly lower than the birth weights of children born to non-smoking mothers [12]. Subsequently, childhood BMI at each checkup age significantly increased but only among male children born to smoking mothers [12]. Furthermore, it was observed that this increase continued after 3 years of age (Fig. 2.2) [12].

Next, Zheng et al. described gender-based height growth patterns in Japanese school-aged children using a multilevel analysis, as determining standard pubertal growth patterns using longitudinal anthropometric measures is important in growth assessment [17]. Height was similar between genders at 6.5–9.5 years of age [17]. Then, girls grew faster and were taller than boys at 10.5–11.5 years of age [17]. Subsequently, boys caught up and exceeded girls' heights starting at age 12.5 [17]. Height gain trajectories showed that the girls' annual height gains increased slowly and peaked from 9.5 to 11.5 years of age, while boys' height gains declined slightly at first and peaked at 11.5–12.5 years of age [17]. The gender-based differences in height gains were significant from 7.5 to 14.5 years of age ($p < 0.0001$) [17]. Growth rate and height gain trajectories were similar between genders, although pubertal growth spurts were observed earlier in girls than in boys [17]. Moreover, Wei et al.

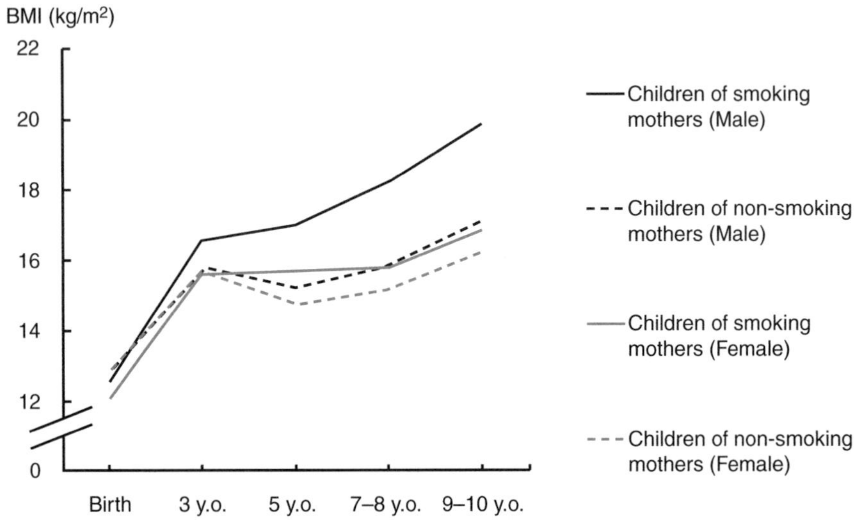

Fig. 2.2 Children's body mass index trajectories by maternal smoking status during pregnancy, calculated by individual growth analysis (original data: Suzuki, 2015 [8])

examined the differences in growth patterns during adolescence between overweight/obese and non-overweight children in Japan [18]. Overweight/obese girls grew taller in the first half period, reached their peak height gain about a year earlier than non-overweight girls did, and experienced an earlier decrease in height gain [18]. Similarly, it was initially observed that overweight/obese boys gained more height than non-overweight boys did [18]. Additionally, non-overweight boys maintained a higher rate of height gain from the age of peak height gain, although the age of peak height gain did not differ between the two groups [18].

Finally, we conducted a kind of pathway analysis between maternal smoking during pregnancy and infancy growth. As a result, maternal smoking during pregnancy contributed to lower birth weight as well as previous findings [25]. In addition, lower birth weight contributed significantly to rapid infancy growth. Maternal smoking during pregnancy was also related to infant growth through breastfeeding status during the first 3 months [25]. The indirect standardized effect of maternal smoking through the three pathways was 0.04 [25]. In addition, maternal smoking was also directly linked to rapid infancy growth. The standardized direct effect was 0.06 ($p = 0.002$) [25]. Taking all the pathways into account, the standardized total effect of maternal smoking on infancy growth was 0.11 [25]. It was suggested that maternal smoking during pregnancy may both indirectly, through birth weight, breastfeeding status, and directly influence rapid infant growth; further, other pathways have not yet been identified (Fig. 2.3).

Because this cohort study is conducted only in a rural area in Japan, there are some limitations. For example, it is necessary to consider statistical power because, as mentioned above, the number of annual births is relatively small. In addition, there are few clinical information because this study was community-based.

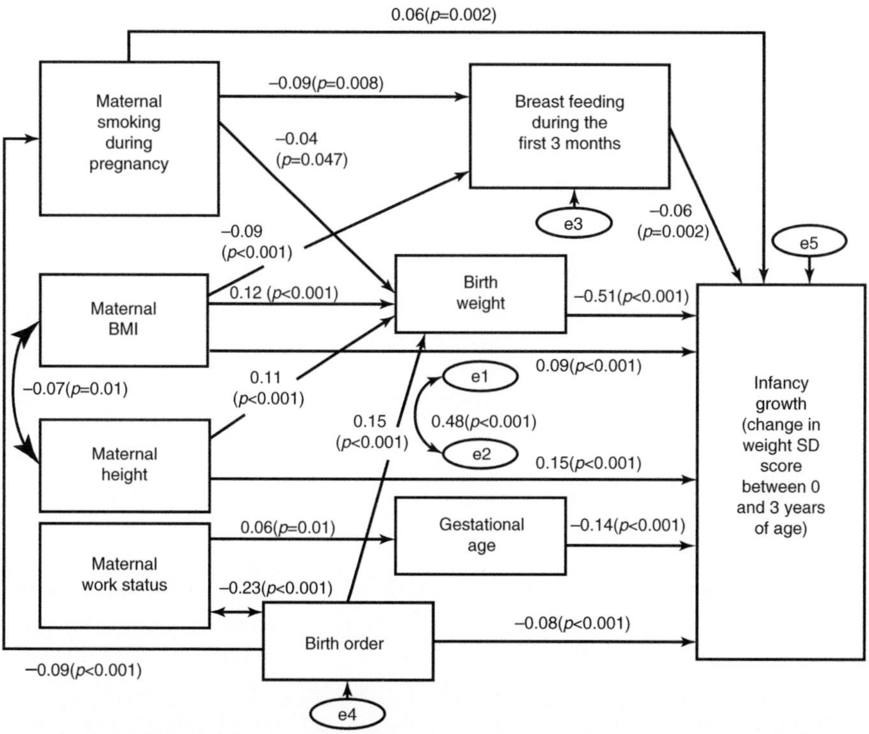

Fig. 2.3 Standardized pathways between maternal smoking during pregnancy and infancy growth determined using exploratory methods (original data: Zheng et al., 2015 [25])

However, the issue about selection bias might be small because the follow-up rate is approximately 80% at 10 years of age [12]. Thus, it might be important to establish some evidence about DOHaD from this kind of small community-based cohort study because the feasibility might be relatively higher than the large cohort study like JECS.

2.3 Longitudinal Surveys of Newborns in the Twenty-First Century (2001 Cohort and 2010 Cohort)

2.3.1 The Overview of Longitudinal Surveys of Babies Born in the Twenty-First Century

This national representative prospective cohort studies were conducted by the Ministry of Health, Labour and Welfare. The overview of the survey was described in some related articles [26–28]. First, children born between January 10 and 17,

2001, and between July 10 and 17, 2001, and their fathers and mothers were recruited for the 2001 survey based on the information of birth registration data in vital statistics ($n = 53{,}575$). On the other hand, children born between May 10 and 24, 2010 were recruited for the 2010 survey in the same method for the 2001 survey ($n = 43{,}767$). These data were linked with the birth registration record data of vital statistics. A total of 47,015 and 38,554 respondents participated in the first survey which was conducted in 2001 and 2010, respectively.

In the first survey, guardian, household, employment (including child care leave), working hours, sharing in household chores and child rearing by parents, housing conditions, efforts and attempts in child rearing, advantages of having the baby, disadvantages of having the baby, worries and anxieties about child rearing, breastfeeding, income, maternal smoking status after delivery (6 months later), and maternal and paternal educational backgrounds (the first follow-up survey) were collected by the questionnaire. At each annual survey, the contents of questionnaires were slightly changed based on childhood growth and development. On the other hand, sex of the children, birth weight, gestational weeks, birth order, nationality of mothers and fathers, and maternal age at their delivery were collected by birth registration data.

All respondents consented to the purpose of these surveys described by the Ministry of Health, Labour and Welfare. Moreover, the data of this survey was completely anonymized and de-identified by the government when the data was provided to the researchers who were permitted to use by the government.

Some of the results of each survey were described in the website of the Ministry of Health, Labour and Welfare [6].

2.3.2 Some Findings Related to DOHaD from Longitudinal Survey of Newborns in the Twenty-First Century

As mentioned above, because it is essential to be obtained permission to use the data of survey by the government, the number of articles by using the data of this survey was relatively limited. In addition, it is relatively difficult to examine the effect of factors during fetal period on childhood growth and development because these surveys were commenced at birth. However, there were some valuable findings from the surveys.

First, because it has been suggested that socioeconomic status was associated with healthy lifestyle, such as nutrition, physical activity, and smoking status [29–31], socioeconomic status might be an important factor which is associated with DOHaD. Fujiwara et al. examined the impact of income inequality and parental socioeconomic status on several birth outcomes [26]. It was observed that higher prefectural income inequality was associated with z-score of birth weight for gestational age, but not with only gestational age in multilevel analysis [26]. In addition, there was significant association between parental educational level and the z-score of birth weight for gestational age and small-for-gestational-age status [26].

Next, regarding childhood physical growth, Franchetti and Ide described the trajectories of childhood BMI, especially focused on adiposity rebound, and examined the association between sociodemographic and lifestyle factors and childhood growth [27]. As a result, after controlling for sex, obese children had a 48.5% higher hazard to experience AR than nonobese children by Cox's proportional hazards model [27]. In addition, the difference in BMI transition between obese and nonobese children was also captured by description of trajectories [27]. Regarding the sociodemographic and lifestyle factors, children who had a longer gestational period were likely to be lower BMI [27]. On the other hand, children who received parental care from nonfamily members were likely to be higher BMI [27].

Finally, Higa Diez et al. described the association between preterm birth and childhood behavioral outcomes (three attention problems and four delinquent/aggressive behaviors) at 8 years of age [28]. In logistic regression model, positive associations were observed between preterm birth (<37 weeks) and adverse behavioral outcomes compared with full-term birth (39–41 weeks) [28]. For attention problems, it was suggested that preterm birth was significantly associated with "inability to wait for his/her turn" [28]. It was suggested that preterm birth is significantly associated with increasing risk of behavioral problems related to attention and delinquent/aggressive behavior at 8 years old [28].

Although these results were only based on the survey of 2001 cohort, it is possible to use the data of 2010 cohort which is almost similar items to the survey of 2001 cohort. Therefore, it might be possible to compare the childhood outcomes or the associations between sociodemographic and lifestyle factors and these outcomes between two surveys. In the future, some valuable findings related to DOHaD, especially the effect of childhood lifestyle and environment, during early infancy period might be produced.

2.4 Japan Environment and Children's Study (JECS)

2.4.1 The Overview of Japan Environment and Children's Study (JECS)

For JECS, pregnant women were recruited between January 31, 2011 and March 31, 2014. Eligibility criteria for participants (expectant mothers) were as follows: (1) residing in the study area at the time of recruitment, (2) expected delivery date after August 1, 2011, and (3) capable of comprehending the Japanese language and completing the self-administered questionnaire. Individuals residing outside the study area who attended cooperating healthcare providers within the study area were excluded from the study. Details of the JECS project have been described in a previous article [7]. The response rate of JECS was about 79% [32]. Because the recruitment period was relatively long, there were some datasets which included not only all participants but also a part of participants. For example, we used the first fixed dataset named as "jecs-ag-ai-20131008 dataset," which was released in October 2013. Detail of this dataset was published previously [33]. This dataset consisted of information on 9369 singleton infants born before December 31, 2011 [34]. The mean age and standard deviation (SD) of participants in this dataset was 31.0 ± 5.0 years [34]. The mean gestational duration and SD at their pregnancy registration was 108.6 ± 42.7 days [34]. Recently, the complete dataset at birth has been released and distributed to the JECS researchers.

The JECS protocol was approved by the Institutional Review Board on epidemiological studies of the Ministry of the Environment and the Ethics Committees of all participating institutions: the National Institute for Environmental Studies which leads the JECS, the National Center for Child Health and Development, Hokkaido University, Sapporo Medical University, Asahikawa Medical College, Japanese Red Cross Hokkaido College of Nursing, Tohoku University, Fukushima Medical University, Chiba University, Yokohama City University, University of Yamanashi, Shinshu University, University of Toyama, Nagoya City University, Kyoto University, Doshisha University, Osaka University, Osaka Medical Center and Research Institute for Maternal and Child Health, Hyogo College of Medicine, Tottori University, Kochi University, University of Occupational and Environmental Health, Kyushu University, Kumamoto University, University of Miyazaki, and University of the Ryukyus. The JECS was conducted in accordance with the Helsinki Declaration and other nationally valid regulations and guidelines.

Information of mothers and their partners during the mothers' pregnancy was collected by questionnaire during the first and second trimesters of pregnancy [7]. The questionnaire included questions about lifestyle factors (stress levels, diet, smoking habits, alcohol consumption, physical activity, sleeping patterns, infections, and medication), SES, and physical environment (heat, ionizing radiation, housing conditions, and neighborhood) [7]. Maternal anthropometric data before pregnancy and data on maternal weight gain during pregnancy and complications before and during pregnancy including pregnancy-induced hypertension (PIH), diabetes mellitus (DM) and gestational diabetes mellitus (GDM), history of previous pregnancy, sex of infants, birth order, and perinatal outcomes such as birth weight and gestational duration were also collected from medical records, which were provided by their obstetricians [7].

2.4.2 Some Findings Related to DOHaD from JECS

Because JECS is relatively new birth cohort study, only few articles which used the fixed data were published. Moreover, it is difficult to confirm childhood outcomes after birth because it took only approximately 1 year after the final birth of participants. In this section, I introduce two articles which used the fixed dataset of JECS.

First, although there were a lot of articles to describe the association between maternal smoking during pregnancy and birthweight, to the best of our knowledge, there have been no large nationwide population-based epidemiological studies examining the association that simultaneously controlled for clinical information, SES, pregestational BMI, and maternal weight gain during pregnancy. Thus, we described the association between maternal smoking status during pregnancy and birth weight while taking these confounding factors into consideration [34]. Our analysis utilized the first fixed dataset from JECS. After controlling for potential confounding factors, maternal smoking status during pregnancy was significantly associated with birth weight [34]. There was a significant difference in birth weight between NS and SM for both male and female infants (Table 2.1: male infants, 3096.2 g (Never-smokers: NS) vs. 2959.8 g (Current smokers: SM) [$p < 0.001$]; female infants, 3018.2 g (NS) vs. 2893.7 g (SM) [$p < 0.001$]) [34]. This study provides valuable evidence to support the importance of cessation of maternal smoking before and during pregnancy.

Next, although it has been suggested that severe nausea and vomiting in early pregnancy (NVP) and hyperemesis gravidarum (HG), which is an extreme form of NVP, were associated with weight loss, there is no clear consensus on the association HG and NVP and fetal growth. Thus, Morokuma et al. examined the association between HG and NVP and small-for-gestational-age (SGA) using data of JECS [35]. As a result, the risk ratios of SGA birth (95% confidence interval) for mothers with severe NVP and those with HG were 0.86 (0.62–1.19) and 0.81 (0.39–1.66), respectively [35]. The results suggested that neither severe NVP nor HG was associated with increased risk for SGA birth.

In conclusion, regarding DOHaD, it is important to estimate fetal environment including environmental and maternal lifestyle factors and its effects on fetal and childhood growth and development. Although JECS is relatively new study, there is some strength as a nationwide birth cohort study. In the future, a lot of valuable findings which might contribute to describe and clarify the mechanism of DOHaD could be developed.

2.5 An Example of the Study Using Birth Registration Data (Vital Statistics): Effects of the Great East Japan Earthquake on Secondary Sex Ratio (SSR) and Perinatal Outcomes

2.5.1 Birth Registration Data (Vital Statistics)

In Japan, every birth must be registered by law. These data were anonymously provided under the Statistics Act in Japan. These data contain the birthplace, birth date, sex of children, birth weight, gestational age, parity, and ages of the father and mother. Except for the ages of the parents, the obstetrician who attended the birth provided this information on the birth certificate. It was not compulsory to obtain permission to use their birth registration data in the study from the participants because it is available for researchers to use the birth registration data with permission from the Ministry of Health, Labour and Welfare under the Statistics Act in Japan.

Table 2.1 Crude and Adjusted mean birth weight in male and female infants without preterm birth (original data: Suzuki et al., 2016 [34])

Smoking status during early pregnancy	Male					Female				
	Crude mean birth weight (g)	Standard error	Adjusted mean birth weight (g)[a]	Standard error	*p*-value[b]	Crude mean birth weight (g)	Standard error	Adjusted mean birth weight (g)[a]	Standard error	*p*-value[b]
Never-smokers (NS)	3102.6	8.3	3141.8	17.5		3007.7	8.2	3055.5	16.4	
Ex-smokers who quit before pregancy (QSB)	3110.6	12.1	3133.8	19.2	0.9	3031.6	12.3	3069.2	18.2	0.6
Ex-smokers who quit during early pregnancy (QSD)	3116.9	15.5	3109.7	21.0	0.2	2999.7	16.8	3021.1	20.7	0.14
Current smokers (SM)	2994.1	26.3	3004.6	28.4	<0.001	2875.2	24.7	2928.0	28.2	<0.001

[a]Adjusted for partners' smoking status, annual household income, birth order of children, PIH, DM/GDM, maternal weight before pregnancy, maternal weight gain during pregnancy, maternal age group at delivery and gestational duration calculated by least squares mean adjustment
[b]*p*-value was calculated using Dunnett's test by least squares mean adjustment

2.5.2 The Study Using Birth Registration Data Related to DOHaD

The effect of natural disasters such as earthquake on perinatal outcomes has been previously examined. However, previous studies had certain limitations. For example, although an effect of seasonality may be noted for SSR [36–38] or preterm births [39], none of the above studies strictly adjusted for seasonal changes in perinatal outcomes. Furthermore, when individual data was used for analysis, the sample size of the study was relatively small, while when the number of subjects was large, these studies were designed as ecological studies. Thus, it might be difficult to conclude the causal association between natural disasters and perinatal outcomes. On 11 March 2011, a huge earthquake occurred in East Japan, called the Great East Japan Earthquake. Subsequently, a massive tsunami struck the area, and millions of people were affected by this earthquake and tsunami. This earthquake was determined to be the most severe natural disaster in Japan in recorded history [40]. We examined the effects of the Great East Japan Earthquake on SSR, birth weight, and gestational duration in weeks using individual birth registration data in the most severely affected prefectures and other prefectures in Japan [41].

Individual birth registration data from the vital statistics of Japan between March 2010 and March 2012 were used for this study [41]. To examine the effect of the earthquake on SSR and perinatal outcomes, we compared the following two groups. Pregnant women who experienced the earthquake at 4–36 weeks of gestation were categorized according to their gestational period as of 11 March 2011, as follows: gestational weeks 4–11, 12–19, 20–27, and 28–36 (2011 group, $n = 679{,}131$) [41]. Similarly, pregnant women who did not experience the earthquake were categorized according to their gestational period as of 11 March 2010 and used as controls (2010 group, $n = 688{,}479$) [41].

As a result, in the extremely affected region, the SSR among women at 4–11 weeks of gestation significantly declined in the 2011 group as compared with the 2010 group (Table 2.2: 49.8% vs. 52.1%, $p = 0.009$) [41]. In the extremely affected region, women who experienced the earthquake at 28–36 weeks of gestation were likely to deliver infants with significantly lower birth weights [41]. These results suggested that the SSR declined among women who experienced the earthquake during early pregnancy, particularly in the extremely affected region. However, no apparent negative effect of the earthquake on perinatal outcomes was observed.

From the view of public health, the effect of disaster on perinatal and childhood outcomes might be important. In addition, regarding DOHaD, this kind of large disaster might be an important factor which is associated with fetal and early childhood environment. Therefore, it is important to examine the effect of some environmental factors like disaster on birth outcomes by using the public data like vital statistics.

Table 2.2 Comparison of secondary sex ratio (SSR) of all singleton babies between 2010 group and 2011 group in each gestational period category and region (original data: Suzuki et al., 2016 [41])

Gestational weeks	4–11 weeks			12–19 weeks			20–27 weeks			28–36 weeks		
	Total	Male	*p**	Total	Male	*p*	Total	Male	*p*	Total	Male	*p*
Extremely affected region												
2010 group	6798	3541 52.1	0.009	7082	3680 52.0	0.66	6948	3499 50.4	0.07	7518	3863 51.4	0.07
2011 group	6618	3298 49.8		6716	3465 51.6		6649	3450 51.9		7223	3604 49.9	
Moderately affected region												
2010 group	66,757	34,155 51.2	0.97	65,525	33,949 51.8	0.86	65,018	33,251 51.1	0.28	68,824	35,380 51.4	0.61
2011 group	65,137	33,320 51.2		64,947	33,617 51.8		63,721	32,780 51.4		67,872	34,798 51.3	
Slightly or unaffected region												
2010 group	94,792	48,980 51.7	0.0011	94,700	48,466 51.2	0.43	92,986	48,127 51.8	0.21	99,176	51,149 51.6	0.48
2011 group	93,363	47,541 50.9		94,709	48,641 51.4		91,825	47,257 51.5		98,359	50,573 51.4	

**p values were calculated by Chi-square test*

2.6 Conclusion

In Japan, there are some population-based birth cohort studies, and these studies established the findings related to DOHaD. These population-based DOHaD evidences could directly apply to public health activity not only in local community but also nationwide level. In addition, some previous findings might be valuable to clarify the mechanisms of DOHaD although some epidemiological limitations existed. In the future, it is expected that a lot of scientific evidences will be produced from these cohort studies.

Acknowledgment I thank the participants of these studies, the JECS staff and the collaborating hospitals and clinics, the staff of the Administrative Office of Koshu City and current and former members of the Department Health Sciences and the Center for Birth Cohort Studies, University of Yamanashi.

References

1. Swanson JM, et al. Developmental origins of health and disease: environmental exposures. Semin Reprod Med. 2009;27(5):391–402.
2. Phillips DI. Insulin resistance as a programmed response to fetal undernutrition. Diabetologia. 1996;39(9):1119–22.
3. Eriksson JG, et al. Early adiposity rebound in childhood and risk of Type 2 diabetes in adult life. Diabetologia. 2003;46(2):190–4.
4. Bhargava SK, et al. Relation of serial changes in childhood body-mass index to impaired glucose tolerance in young adulthood. N Engl J Med. 2004;350(9):865–75.
5. Barker DJ, et al. Trajectories of growth among children who have coronary events as adults. N Engl J Med. 2005;353(17):1802–9.
6. Ministry of Health, Labour and Welfare. Longitudinal survey of newborns in the 21st century. 2016. http://www.mhlw.go.jp/english/database/db-hw/vs03.html. Accessed 30 Dec 2016.
7. Kawamoto T, et al. Rationale and study design of the Japan environment and children's study (JECS). BMC Public Health. 2014;14:25.
8. Suzuki K. Longitudinal analyses of childhood growth: evidence from Project Koshu. J Epidemiol. 2015;25(1):2–7.
9. Mizutani T, et al. Association of maternal lifestyles including smoking during pregnancy with childhood obesity. Obesity. 2007;15(12):3133–9.
10. Suzuki K, et al. Is maternal smoking during pregnancy a risk factor for all low birth weight infants? J Epidemiol. 2008;18(3):89–96.
11. Suzuki K, et al. The association between maternal smoking during pregnancy and childhood obesity persists to the age of 9-10 years. J Epidemiol. 2009;19(3):136–42.
12. Suzuki K, et al. Gender differences in the association between maternal smoking during pregnancy and childhood growth trajectories: multi-level analysis. Int J Obes (Lond). 2011;35(1):53–9.
13. Suzuki K, et al. Maternal smoking during pregnancy and childhood growth trajectory: a random effects regression analysis. J Epidemiol. 2012;22(2):175–8.
14. Suzuki K, et al. Differences in the effect of maternal smoking during pregnancy for childhood overweight before and after 5 years of age. J Obstet Gynaecol Res. 2013;39(5):914–21.
15. Suzuki K, et al. Effect of maternal smoking cessation before and during early pregnancy on fetal and childhood growth. J Epidemiol. 2014;24(1):60–6.

16. Suzuki K, et al. Recent trends in the prevalence of and factors associated with maternal smoking during pregnancy in Japan. J Obstet Gynaecol Res. 2010;36(4):745–50.
17. Zheng W, et al. Gender-based differences in longitudinal height gain and growth rate changes in Japanese school-aged children: a multilevel analysis. J Epidemiol. 2013;23(4):275–9.
18. Zheng W, et al. Adolescent growth in overweight and non-overweight children in Japan: a multilevel analysis. Paediatr Perinat Epidemiol. 2014;28(3):263–9.
19. Conter V, et al. Weight growth in infants born to mothers who smoked during pregnancy. BMJ. 1995;310(6982):768–71.
20. Chiolero A, et al. Association between maternal smoking and low birth weight in Switzerland: the EDEN study. Swiss Med Wkly. 2005;135(35–36):525–30.
21. Heaman M, et al. Risk factors for preterm birth and small-for-gestational-age births among Canadian women. Paediatr Perinat Epidemiol. 2013;27(1):54–61.
22. Reeves S, Bernstein I. Effects of maternal tobacco-smoke exposure on fetal growth and neonatal size. Expert Rev Obstet Gynecol. 2008;3(6):719–30.
23. Barker DJ. Mothers, babies, and disease in later life. London: BMJ Publishing; 1994.
24. Twisk JWR. Applied multilevel analysis. New York: Cambridge University Press; 2006.
25. Zheng W, et al. Maternal smoking during pregnancy and infancy growth: a covariance structure analysis. J Epidemiol. 2015;25(1):44–9.
26. Fujiwara T, et al. Income inequality, parental socioeconomic status, and birth outcomes in Japan. Am J Epidemiol. 2013;177(10):1042–52.
27. Franchetti Y, Ide H. Socio-demographic and lifestyle factors for child's physical growth and adiposity rebound of Japanese children: a longitudinal study of the 21st century longitudinal survey in newborns. BMC Public Health. 2014;14:334. https://doi.org/10.1186/1471-2458-14-334.
28. Higa Diez M, et al. Preterm birth and behavioural outcomes at 8 years of age: a nationwide survey in Japan. Arch Dis Child. 2016;101(4):338–43.
29. Fukuda Y, et al. Accumulation of health risk behaviours is associated with lower socioeconomic status and women's urban residence: a multilevel analysis in Japan. BMC Public Health. 2005;5:53.
30. Takeuchi K, et al. Community-level socioeconomic status and parental smoking in Japan. Soc Sci Med. 2012;75(4):747–51.
31. Nakamura S, et al. Association of household income and education with eating behaviors in Japanese adults: a cross-sectional study. BMC Public Health. 2016;16:61. https://doi.org/10.1186/s12889-016-2748-z.
32. Ministry of the Environment. Japan Environment and Children's Study. 2015. http://www.env.go.jp/chemi/ceh/press/data/seminar150119_1.pdf. Accessed 11 Aug 2015.
33. Michikawa T, Nitta H, Nakayama SF, et al. The Japan Environment and Children's Study (JECS): a preliminary report on selected characteristics of approximately 10 000 pregnant women recruited during the first year of the study. J Epidemiol. 2015;25:452–8.
34. Suzuki K, et al. Association between maternal smoking during pregnancy and birth weight: an appropriately adjusted model from the Japan Environment and Children's Study. J Epidemiol. 2016;26(7):371–7.
35. Morokuma S, et al. Relationship between hyperemesis gravidarum and small-for-gestational-age in the Japanese population: the Japan Environment and Children's Study (JECS). BMC Pregnancy Childbirth. 2016;16:247. https://doi.org/10.1186/s12884-016-1041-6.
36. James WH. Interpregnancy intervals, high maternal age and seasonal effects on the human sex ratio. Hum Reprod. 1996;11(1):7–8.
37. Lerchl A. Seasonality of sex ratio in Germany. Hum Reprod. 1998;13(5):1401–2.
38. Melnikov VN, et al. Seasonality bias in adverse pregnancy outcomes in Siberia. Alaska Med. 2007;49(2 Suppl):218–20.
39. Currie J, Schwandt H. Within-mother analysis of seasonal patterns in health at birth. Proc Natl Acad Sci U S A. 2013;110(30):12265–70.
40. Geller R. Shake-up time for Japanese seismology. Nature. 2011;472(7344):407–9.
41. Suzuki K, et al. Effects of the great East Japan earthquake on secondary sex ratio and perinatal outcomes. J Epidemiol. 2016;26(2):76–83.

Chapter 3
DOHaD Interventions: Opportunities During Adolescence and the Periconceptional Period

Jacquie Bay, Delaney Yaqona, and Masahito Oyamada

Abstract Collective evidence underpinning the Developmental Origins of Health and Disease (DOHaD) hypothesis demonstrates that interventions to improve the nutritional environment during early life offer an important opportunity for primary prevention of DOHaD-related noncommunicable diseases (NCDs). This evidence has led to important programs targeting pregnancy and early childhood. However, addressing the full potential of the DOHaD paradigm also requires consideration of the periconceptional period, and therefore health behaviors prior to pregnancy and parenthood, alongside the complex array of personal and societal factors influencing these behaviors. Therefore, adolescence, the life stage during which cognitive, psychosocial, and lifestyle behaviors that persist into adulthood are formed, should be a key DOHaD intervention point. Schools and tertiary institutions play a major role in the lives of adolescents, supporting the development of capabilities associated with engaged citizenship including scientific and health literacies and key life competencies. Providing young people who are developing these capabilities with opportunities to examine evidence about NCD risk and prevention can empower adolescents to engage in development of and/or participation in evidence-based actions that can contribute toward interrupting the transgenerational conditioning/programming of NCD vulnerability. Realizing the potential of interventions that target the adolescent life stage requires effective cross-sectoral partnerships between education, science, and public health. Education should be a key partner, bringing important expertise alongside that of health and science to facilitate the task of the translation of DOHaD evidence to adolescents within community settings.

J. Bay (✉)
Liggins Institute, University of Auckland, Auckland, New Zealand
e-mail: j.bay@auckland.ac.nz

D. Yaqona
Nukutere College, Rarotonga, Cook Islands

M. Oyamada
Department of Food Science and Human Nutrition, Fuji Women's University, Sapporo, Hokkaido, Japan
e-mail: oyamada@fujijoshi.ac.jp

F. Sata et al. (eds.), *Pre-emptive Medicine: Public Health Aspects of Developmental Origins of Health and Disease*, Current Topics in Environmental Health and Preventive Medicine, https://doi.org/10.1007/978-981-13-2194-8_3

Keywords Adolescent · Periconceptional · Primary NCD risk · Multi-sectoral · Education

Abbreviations

CBPR	Community-based participatory research
DOHaD	Developmental Origins of Health and Disease
ECHO	Commission on Ending Childhood Obesity
NCD	Noncommunicable disease
PE	Physical education
SIDS	Small Island Developing States
WHO	World Health Organization

3.1 Introduction

Evidence from the field of Developmental Origins of Health and Disease (DOHaD) has highlighted biological mechanisms underpinning the intergenerational nature of noncommunicable disease (NCD) risk. It is now understood that early-life environmental exposures contribute to vulnerability *toward* a wide range of adverse conditions spanning the life-course. These include neurocognitive developmental challenges, overweight, obesity, and NCDs ranging from metabolic and cardiovascular diseases to musculoskeletal, allergic, and mental health conditions [1]. Investigation of the mechanisms underpinning these observations has demonstrated that environmentally mediated epigenetic modifications result in the latent phenotypic influences that are associated with increased NCD risk [2]. This evidence has highlighted previously untapped primary prevention opportunities that could contribute toward interrupting the intergenerational cycle of NCD risk. The potential of such interventions is increasingly recognized as a valid NCD risk reduction strategy by global agencies [3]. The influence of socio-ecological factors on environmental exposures central to the DOHaD paradigm should always be considered in conjunction with the biological evidence.

The window during which environmental exposures may influence later-life health stretches from preconception to early childhood and adolescence [1]. While both nutritional and non-nutritional exposures are important, for this chapter we will focus on nutritional exposures. Both undernutrition and obesogenic early-life environments have been shown to be associated with adverse later-life health outcomes [4], some of which may be indicated by changes as early as childhood [5]. Additionally, maternal pre-pregnancy obesity and excessive gestational weight gain are associated with adverse short-term maternal and offspring impacts as well as obesity-related adverse later-life outcomes in offspring [6]. Evolving from this evidence has been extensive discussion of the potential of targeted interventions during pregnancy and early childhood [7, 8]. These are important and should be pursued, particularly if they support parents to understand the long-term importance of good nutrition in early childhood. However, there is strong evidence to suggest that opportunities to change environmental exposures associated with nutritional practices during pregnancy are limited [9–11]. Additionally, once obesity is established, it is extremely difficult to reverse the biological factors that support the ongoing condition in the individual [12]. While evidence emerging from studies of weight loss prior to pregnancy in humans is limited, maternal surgical weight loss approaches appear to be beneficial for the offspring, as does limiting gestational weight gain [13]. However, evidence from animal models suggests that weight loss within the periconceptional period may be associated with negative downstream effects on metabolic health [13]. Therefore, while addressing the impact of poor-quality nutrition, overweight and/or obesity in the mother during the pregnancy is well-founded, it is challenging. Including adolescence alongside pregnancy as a life-stage target for DOHaD interventions offers the opportunity to address nutritional practices and parental overweight/obesity prior to conception. If successful, such interventions support reductions in the impacts of environmental exposures in the periconceptional period and during pregnancy and remove or reduce the need for periconceptional weight loss and the associated potential risks. This chapter examining the potential of DOHaD interventions within the adolescent period is largely based on our previous reviews on this topic [14–16].

3.2 The Opportunity of Adolescence

Adolescence, the period of transition between childhood and adulthood (age 10–19 years), is a life stage of significant change during which life-long cognitive and psychosocial behaviors are established [17, 18]. Many of these behaviors will influence future health, particularly those associated with the development of overweight, obesity, and associated NCDs [19, 20]. Therefore, adolescence is considered an important component of the life-course approach to the prevention of chronic diseases [21–23].

Intervention during adolescence, even when this is significantly distanced from parenthood, provides an important opportunity to address environmental exposures across a wide range of critical and sensitive life stages. These include:

- **Gametogenesis** and the **periconceptional period** during which unfavorable health status in either parent and/or a poor maternal nutritional environment are associated with adverse short- and long-term health consequences for offspring [1, 13, 24, 25]
- **Pregnancy**, during which maternal overnutrition and overweight or obese status are associated with a wide range of adverse obstetric, infant, childhood, and later-life health outcomes [13, 26]; and maternal undernutrition when associated with poor fetal growth leads to a range of irreversible adverse biological and social consequences, and when associated with low birth weight followed by rapid catch-up growth in childhood and adolescence is associated with increased risk of nutrition-related chronic diseases in adulthood [27].

- **Infancy** and **childhood**, where established nutritional practices of the parents influence the nutritional environment of the infant and child [28, 29], impacting current and later-life health.
- **Adolescence**, where personal control over food choices increases [30]; the influence of family food environment on food choices reduces [31] while the influence of peer food practices increases [32]; lifelong nutritional and related lifestyle practices are established [33]; and the opportunity exists to promote food and lifestyle choices that reduce weight gain [34] either before overweight and obesity are established or before obesity reaches the point where biologically it will be very difficult to reverse [12].

The period of adolescence is almost universally dominated by formal education, encompassing schooling, followed for many by apprenticeships and/or tertiary training or education. The social structures within which formal education occurs support in-depth engagement with adolescents. In the schooling sector, this also engages the family/caregivers. Therefore, it is not surprising that recommendations regarding interventions associated with promoting adolescent health have a focus on multi-sectoral approaches and highlight opportunities associated with schooling [35–37]. Other social structures including religious organizations (e.g., churches, mosques, and synagogues), sporting, service, arts, and cultural clubs also support adolescent development and offer important opportunities that contribute to the development of well-being. While our focus is on the role of the formal education sector, aspects of the approaches described may also be applicable to informal education and community settings.

3.3 Schools as a Setting

Many school-based health-promotion interventions have not been particularly effective [38]. Lack of connection to the core mission of schools has been identified as a key issue associated with poor outcomes [39]. This suggests that program design has failed to attend to the need for shared vision that is inclusive of all participating sectors, known to be the most critical success factor associated with multi-sectoral partnerships [40]. Heterogeneity of impact is a further challenge that is commonly identified as problematic when evidence-informed health policies and practices are applied to school-based health promotion [41]. In education, it is known that failure to address diversity within and between schools magnifies achievement variance (psychosocial and academic) [42]. Heterogeneity of effect in school-based health promotion is likely to be associated with lack of connection to core principles of pedagogy and practice associated with recognizing and addressing diversity. This issue may be addressed through collaborative input of educators into school-based health-promotion design.

Thus, to achieve the potential of DOHaD interventions that support the opportunities offered by the development of positive health-related practices during adolescence, attention must be paid to developing multi-sectoral and community-based participatory research (CBPR) approaches that engage with school communities. Interventions must connect to core goals in education as well as health and science and recognize the important role that each school community has in adapting and sustaining programs that are specific to their setting [14, 16]. CBPR approaches are optimal; recognizing that knowledge and expertise from within the community in which the intervention is occurring should have a central role in determining the nature of the research question, intervention tools, evaluation methods, and interpretation [43]. Such approaches support the potential for interventions to not only link to core national education goals but also to specific goals within each school community. This ensures that interventions can be enacted *within* the core business of the school. These approaches address issues of sustainability while simultaneously facilitating the development of capabilities in youth that support action-oriented adolescent empowerment associated with engaged citizenship [15].

It was therefore encouraging to see a shift in the thinking of the World Health Organization (WHO) in the recently published Report from the Commission on Ending Childhood Obesity (ECHO) that explicitly identified the importance of engagement and consultation with the education sector to ensure educational rigor in intervention design and enable interventions to be embedded in mainstream curricula [37].

3.3.1 Understanding the Core Mission of Schools

Modern education systems are concerned with holistic development that "prepares young people to participate as critically engaged citizens and lifelong-learners able to negotiate present realities as well as futures that we cannot predict [14]." To achieve this schools are equipped with structures that support cognitive, physical, and psychosocial (mental, emotional, social, and spiritual) development as well as pastoral care. This holistic approach has seen a shift away from silo-based didactic education of the mid-twentieth century toward integrated educational approaches that support adolescents to develop capabilities (knowledge, skills, attitudes, and values) seen as being essential for living and thriving in the twenty-first century [44]. These extend learning to include cultivation of skills and dispositions associated with critical and creative thinking, collaboration, leadership, entrepreneurship, and active participation in society [45]. This does not preclude learning associated with mastering content knowledge. Rather it stretches adolescents to develop capabilities that enable them to apply academic content knowledge to life situations, including complex contemporary problems such as the NCD epidemic, global warming, poverty, and political instability [45, 46]. This approach to education supports the development of critically engaged citizenship, a way of being that is associated with questioning, seeking evidence and understanding, assessing multiple perspectives, and taking considered actions that are mindful of the complexity of the challenges and opportunities facing modern societies. Thus, the NCD epidemic and DOHaD provide a broad array of contexts that can be utilized by teachers in the delivery of education programs that support curricula goals related to capability development across and within traditional learning disciplines [14].

3.3.2 Capabilities That Enable Adolescents as Critically Engaged Citizens

Capabilities developed during adolescence should enable critically engaged participation in all aspects of society. In the context of the NCD epidemic, critically engaged citizens will interact with the issue of NCD risk, burden, and impact. They will question the status quo (particularly when this is associated with inequities) and seek out and examine evidence from multiple perspectives. This process leads to active participation in evidence-based actions at personal, family, and potentially community/societal level that address challenges associated with the issue. Specific capabilities required to achieve engaged citizenship related to issues associated with NCDs/DOHaD include scientific, health, environmental, and sociological literacies, as well as key competencies and self-efficacy [15]. Literacies in this context refer to the ability to seek out, engage with, examine, and use evidence to make informed decisions. For example, scientific literacy is associated with attaining and using relevant knowledge, skills, attitudes, and values that enable individuals and/or groups to engage with and act upon scientific evidence relating to everyday experiences as well as complex, open-ended issues. Because of the complex and value-laden nature of issues related to the NCD epidemic, education programs should also facilitate understanding of the need to integrate multiple perspectives from the sciences, humanities, and arts, along with social and ethical perspectives into consideration when approaching decision-making [47]. This can be challenging but is transformative when it allows young people to identify and use frames of reference outside their current experience that offer the potential to address issues of concern.

Intervention design must take account of the processes via which capability development and behavior setting occur during adolescence. Capability development during adolescence is a component of human development, influenced by complex interactions over time between the individual's personal attributes and the socio-ecological systems within the environment(s) in which they are developing [48]. This emphasizes the nature of human development as a complex adaptive system. As such, capability development is a dynamic process involving a large number of elements interacting in a nonlinear manner with each other and their environment. These elements can be influenced by the system's history as well as its current context and can be disproportionately affected by small changes [49]. Bronfenbrenner's bioecological model of human development, while acknowledging the complex interactions between the individual and both direct and indirect aspects of the environment, emphasizes the strength of influence of the individual's microsystem, being the most proximal layer of interaction that an individual has with their environment and processes within it [50].

The proximal environment of the adolescent is dominated by family, school, peers, and community interactions (actual and virtual). The knowledge, attitudes, and beliefs that are held individually by the adolescent and by social consensus within the environments in which they interact will influence their behavioral development and their potential to develop the habits of mind associated with critically engaged citizenship. There is increasing public awareness of overweight, obesity, and related diseases known to health and science communities as NCDs. Media, politics, public health messaging, and increasing community experience of these issues are contributing to this and reach adolescents through family, school, and community interactions. However, this awareness is dominated by reductionist thinking that places the actions of the individual at the center of the cause of overweight, obesity, and NCDs. In communities ranging from Japan, New Zealand, Pacific Island states, and Europe, very low levels of awareness of life-course perspectives of NCD risk are found in adolescents, parents, young adults, and the public [51–57]. Exposing adolescents to evidence that challenges this reductionist perspective should be a key objective of school-based DOHaD interventions.

3.3.3 Intervention Tools and Frameworks

If teachers are to use NCD-/DOHaD-related contexts to support the development of capabilities as we have described, they need access to learning resources that enable young people to examine evidence relating to NCD risk and incidence, as well as DOHaD observational and mechanistic evidence (Fig. 3.1).

The use of narrative-based pedagogies has been shown to be very effective in supporting young people to explore and act on research evidence [53, 58]. Narrative-based pedagogies are designed to enable learners to engage with the culture of science and develop deeper understanding of the nature of science as a knowledge system [59]. By providing young people with reimaged scientific evidence to explore and interpret [60], students are able to construct understanding of both the process of science and the emergent evidence [61]. This process of constructing understanding is supportive of transformative learning that leads to action taking that can impact not only the young person but also their peers and/or family (Case Study 1).

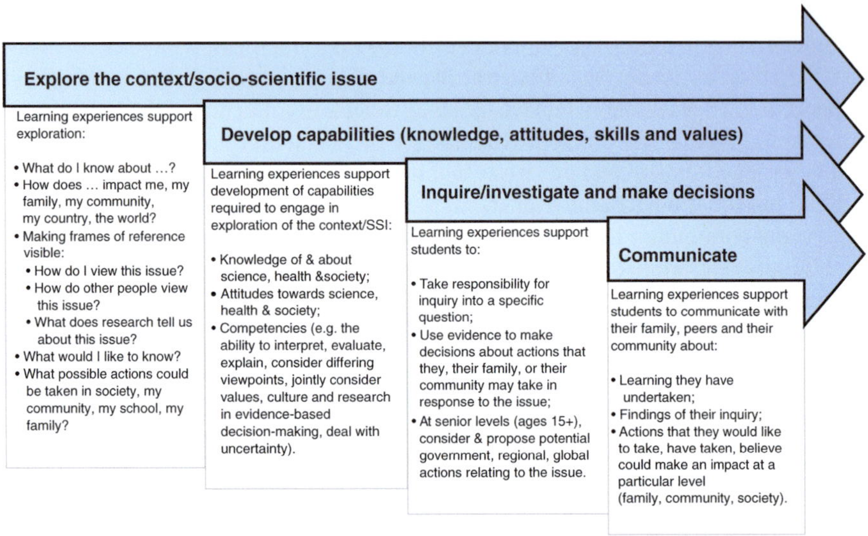

Fig. 3.1 Healthy start to life education for adolescent project learning and teaching module framework [58]

Case Study 1

The Healthy Start to Life Education for Adolescents Project utilizes the trend for contextualization of science education in exploration of socioscientific issues to support development of scientific and health literacy in the context of a life-course approach to NCD risk reduction [52]. Matched pre-post questionnaire evidence demonstrates knowledge, attitude, and behavior (KAB) change, facilitating health-promoting actions that we have demonstrated are sustained in most to 12 months post-intervention [53, 58]. Triangulation with parental data contextualizes aspects of this quantitative evidence. David[1] is a 13-year-old of Pacific Island heritage from a low socioeconomic community in New Zealand. Adult obesity within Pacific peoples in New Zealand is 65% [62]. David's pre-post questionnaire data showed KAB change, including reducing the consumption of deep-fried chips from daily to once per week. Parental interview evidence places this change in context, demonstrating an association with peer relationships.

"There is a local take-away up here … he would always go up after school to get hot chips with his mates. I am so glad that he has actually come away from that. Because he has learnt about diabetes and sugar and fat he has come away from that and he is not doing it" (parent of David (see Footnote 1), 12-week post-intervention interview).

[1] Names have been altered.

Parental data can uncover family-level impact. Questionnaires demonstrated that adolescents had facilitated changes in parental knowledge relating to evidence of the association between early-life nutrition and later-life health ($p < 0.001$), with 72% of parents reporting relevant family-level learning that had occurred during the period of the intervention. Qualitative data provides contextualization of this. Jonah (see Footnote 1) is from the same community as David. His parents spoke of family-level change, as well as reporting that Jonah stopped truanting school during the program.

"He brought the [program] book home and at dinner he told us all about what he has been learning in science about food…..And we talked about that and how it was different to what we were eating…….and we have started eating salads every night since that week. We are proud of him and……he is attending class…. he is really motivated about school" (parents of Jonah, joint 12-week post-intervention interview).

3.3.4 Addressing Gender Equity Issues

DOHaD interventions tend to emphasize adolescent girls and mothers. While this is important, if only females are exposed to programs that support development of understanding of a life-course approach to NCD risk, we cannot expect to change sociocultural norms associated with reductionist thinking regarding NCD cause and/or lack of prioritization of women and children's health and well-being. Behaviors associated with food resources in households are inherently linked to sociocultural norms. In many communities, gender equity issues contribute to the challenges associated with ensuring that adolescent girls and women are empowered to take actions that support well-being. These include simply having full access to available nutritional resources. Incorporating boys and young men into intervention programs is of paramount importance in ensuring that males, through the development of understanding of the importance of nutrition for women and girls, and of their own environment, will be supportive of women's efforts to initiate health-promoting change [63]. While the NCD/DOHaD evidence is weighted strongly toward the role of maternal exposures before and during pregnancy, as noted by Richardson and colleagues [64], public communication that ignores the role of paternal nutrition prior to pregnancy increases the likelihood of "mother at fault" being the overwhelming message heard by society. In addition to the known social influence of males on resources for women and children in many societies, there is clear and growing evidence of the role of paternal preconceptional health in programming/conditioning of later-life health of offspring [25, 65]. Therefore, consideration of gender equity issues and engaging boys *and* men should not be overlooked in the development and implementation of adolescent interventions.

3.3.5 Teachers as Partners in Health Promotion

Teachers from multiple learning disciplines have the potential to play a very valuable role in facilitating action-oriented health promotion. However, this is not the core business of schools facing pressure to meet extensive and growing academic, psychosocial, and pastoral care demands within limited classroom contact time. For teachers to engage in collaborative programs that promote adolescent empowerment regarding life-course NCD risk reduction, they must be provided with appropriate professional development that (a) addresses pedagogical issues while also examining NCD and DOHaD evidence [66, 67] and (b) enables teachers to identify added educational value emerging from program participation (Case Study 2).

Case Study 2

Apii (see Footnote 1) lives in the Cook Islands, a Small Island Developing State (SIDS) in the Pacific with the adult overweight/obesity rates of 91%/72% and type 2 diabetes rates of 26% [68]. At age 13 Apii participated in a Healthy Start to Life Education for Adolescents Program that was co-constructed by his science teacher, working with a team from the Cook Islands Ministries of Health and Education and the Liggins Institute. The program centered on exploration of Cook Islands NCD evidence alongside DOHaD observational and mechanistic evidence. Apii is an engaged student in a mixed ability class with a BMI within the healthy range. Pre-intervention evidence demonstrated that some of his food-related behaviors were not ideal, placing him at increased future NCD risk. Three-month post-intervention data (questionnaire and interview) demonstrated a positive change in relevant food-related behaviors, typical of that demonstrated across intervention cohorts in the precursor program.

In response to the positive cohort-wide educational impact of the program, Apii's science teacher redesigned the following year's learning plan to include a module exploring relevant physiological systems, linking this to the learning goals of the national curriculum. Students were required to research and develop an oral and/or visual presentation examining impacts associated with poor diet in the Cook Islands. Apii (aged 14 years) sought out and presented national-level data on obesity, relating this to NCD risk and determinants of health in the local environment. Using his own data (BMI and lifestyle behaviors), he explored the concept of risk development over time and challenged his peers to examine and change their behaviors, as he explained he had as a result of the previous year's learning program. Assessment of capabilities associated with seeking out, interpreting, and using data to present and act on a justified opinion regarding a socioscientific issue (an achievement objective within the Cook Islands National Curriculum) demonstrated that Apii was now working above the level expected for his age and in relation to his prior academic performance.

3.4 Conclusions: With Not to… the Untapped Potential of Adolescence

Adolescents are frequently represented as "passive participants in social life with little agency in matters concerning them" when in fact they have considerable agency in food practices and actively contribute to and exert power in shaping of food consumption and lifestyle practices [69]. If developed, the potential to harness this agency to drive positive outcomes for adolescents, their families, and their future offspring can be transformational. Achieving this requires investment in multi-sectoral partnerships that recognize that access to scientific evidence is a fundamental human right [70] that is all too frequently ignored.

The purpose of such partnerships must be about empowering adolescents by communicating *with* adolescents and school communities, rather than talking *to* adolescents. This requires resource investment that facilitates the sharing of research evidence in a manner that allows adolescents to construct meaning from and act on evidence in ways that are appropriate to their personal and social context. By collaborating with education and applying modern pedagogy and practice, it is possible to develop innovative interventions that can affect positive change at the level of participating schools, adolescents, and families. Unless such programs are responsive (and hence messy), they will not be meeting the needs of the community in which they are being enacted. This can be challenging as it demands that power in the research relationship is shared and that all participants (scientists, public health professionals, educators, students, and families) are learners. Furthermore, adolescent voices need to be valued in the development of such interventions. We will therefore conclude with an excerpt from a speech given by Jasmine Crosbie, a 19-year-old high school graduate from Auckland, New Zealand, who has participated in such intervention programs since the age of 14 and is also a mother. Jasmine's contribution to a forum in which members of the WHO Commission on Ending Childhood Obesity met with youth from New Zealand schools who had experienced such programs led to her accepting an invitation to present in behalf of youth at the launch of the ECHO report during a side event at the 69th World Health Assembly.

> "*...There are two issues here. Firstly, the environment obviously needs to change. How can young people make healthy food decisions when they are being suffocated by excess unhealthy options in their communities.... Secondly, young people need to be empowered as evidence-based decision makers. Environmental changes without empowerment are not the answer. Young people, just like adults, don't follow rules that they don't understand. We could throw in more fruit and vegetable stores of better quality... ...all to outweigh the unhealthy options. Could do, but the community won't understand! They'll simply head elsewhere for the food they're used to, the food they've been raised around. You may remember being a kid and your parents asking you to do something, you responding with 'why?', and them answering with 'because I said so!' Did you ever do it? No, because you weren't provided with any reasonable explanation of why you should.* ***Young people need to be treated with respect and therefore given the opportunity to explore the issue and evidence and to make decisions based on evidence that work in our context.*** *We not only need to change the obesogenic environment, but education also. I don't believe the classes on healthy eating in*

Health Studies were enough, nor were the P.E lessons. We need to start education around this issue at primary school age, if not before, and in multiple different approved subjects in high school, not just Health and P.E. So to be clear, I do not mean that we would have a few add-on lessons about this. What I am talking about is exploring issues such as obesity, NCDs, diabetes, and life-course evidence in depth within our ordinary subjects like science, social studies, food technology, health and PE, English and maths. ***Because young people ARE interested in issues. We DO care. We DON'T just live in the present. We DO think about our futures and the futures of our families. We are intelligent and we can be the decision makers.*** *May I remind you that the Universal declaration of human rights states that it is the right of every human to "share in scientific advancement and its benefits" So to learn about the life-course approach to NCD risk reduction and the wider societal issues is empowering. As a young mother, that sense of empowerment was huge for me.*"

Jasmine Crosbie, Geneva, May 2016 [71]

References

1. Hanson MA, Gluckman PD. Early developmental conditioning of later health and disease: physiology or pathophysiology? Physiol Rev. 2014;94(4):1027–76.
2. Jiang X. Nutrition in early life, epigenetics, and health. Epigenetics, the environment, and children's health across lifespans. New York: Springer; 2016. p. 135–58.
3. Chestnov O, Hilten MV, McIff C, Kulikov A. Rallying United Nations organizations in the fight against noncommunicable diseases. Bull World Health Organ. 2013;91:623-A.
4. Vickers MH. Developmental programming of the metabolic syndrome—critical windows for intervention. World J Diabetes. 2011;2(9):137–48.
5. Godfrey KM, Sheppard A, Gluckman PD, Lillycrop KA, Burdge GC, McLean C, et al. Epigenetic gene promoter methylation at birth is associated with child's later adiposity. Diabetes. 2011;60(5):1528–34.
6. Patel N, Poston L. Maternal obesity and gestational weight gain as determinants of long-term health. Parental obesity: intergenerational programming and consequences. New York: Springer; 2016. p. 33–56.
7. Balbus JM, Barouki R, Birnbaum LS, Etzel RA, Gluckman PD Sr, Grandjean P, et al. Early-life prevention of non-communicable diseases. Lancet. 2013;381(9860):3–4.
8. Gillman MW. Early infancy—a critical period for development of obesity. J Dev Orig Health Dis. 2010;1(5):292–9.
9. Crozier SR, Robinson SM, Godfrey KM, Cooper C, Inskip HM. Women's dietary patterns change little from before to during pregnancy. J Nutr. 2009;139(10):1956–63.
10. Morton SM, Grant CC, Wall CR, Atatoan Carr PE, Bandara DK, Shmidt JM, et al. Adherence to nutritional guidelines in pregnancy: evidence from the Growing Up in New Zealand birth cohort study. Public Health Nutr. 2014;17(9):1919–29.
11. Kubota K, Itoh H, Tasaka M, Naito H, Fukuoka Y, Muramatsu Kato K, et al. Changes of maternal dietary intake, bodyweight and fetal growth throughout pregnancy in pregnant Japanese women. J Obstet Gynaecol Res. 2013;39(9):1383–90.
12. Blackstone RP. The biology of weight regulation and genetic resetting TM. Obesity. New York: Springer; 2016. p. 41–66.
13. Nicholas LM, McMillen IC. The impact of maternal obesity and weight loss during the periconceptional period on offspring metabolism. In: Green LR, Hester RL, editors. Parental obesity: intergenerational programming and consequences. New York: Springer; 2016. p. 133–61.
14. Bay JL, Vickers MH. Adolescent education: an opportunity to create a Developmental Origins of Health and Disease (DOHaD) circuit breaker. J Dev Orig Health Dis. 2016;7(5):501–4.

15. Bay J, Morton S, Vickers M. Realizing the potential of adolescence to prevent transgenerational conditioning of noncommunicable disease risk: multi-sectoral design frameworks. Healthcare. 2016;4(3):39.
16. Bay JL, Hipkins R, Siddiqi K, Huque R, Dixon R, Shirley D, et al. School-based primary NCD risk reduction: education and public health perspectives. Health Promotion Int. 2017;32(2):369–79.
17. Craigie AM, Lake AA, Kelly SA, Adamson AJ, Mathers JC. Tracking of obesity-related behaviours from childhood to adulthood: a systematic review. Maturitas. 2011;70(3):266–84.
18. Steinberg L. Cognitive and affective development in adolescence. Trends Cogn Sci. 2005;9(2):69–74.
19. Chandola T, Deary IJ, Blane D, Batty GD. Childhood IQ in relation to obesity and weight gain in adult life: the National Child Development (1958) Study. Int J Obes (Lond). 2006;30(9):1422–32.
20. Alberga AS, Sigal RJ, Goldfield G, Prud'homme D, Kenny GP. Overweight and obese teenagers: why is adolescence a critical period? Pediatr Obes. 2012;7(4):261–73.
21. Darnton-Hill I, Nishida C, James WPT. A life course approach to diet, nutrition and the prevention of chronic diseases. Public Health Nutr. 2004;7(1a):101–21.
22. Sawyer SM, Afifi RA, Bearinger LH, Blakemore SJ, Dick B, Ezeh AC, et al. Adolescence: a foundation for future health. Lancet. 2012;379(9826):1630–40.
23. Patton GC, Olsson CA, Skirbekk V, Saffery R, Wlodek ME, Azzopardi PS, et al. Adolescence and the next generation. Nature. 2018;554:458. https://doi.org/10.1038/nature25759.
24. Watkins AJ, Lucas ES, Fleming TP. Impact of the periconceptual environment on the programming of adult disease. J Dev Orig Health Dis. 2010;1(2):87–95.
25. Fullston T, Shehadeh HS, Schjenken JE, McPherson NO, Robertson SA, Zander-Fox D, et al. Paternal obesity and programming of offspring health. Parental obesity: intergenerational programming and consequences. New York: Springer; 2016. p. 105–31.
26. Catalano PM, Ehrenberg HM. Review article: the short- and long-term implications of maternal obesity on the mother and her offspring. BJOG. 2006;113(10):1126–33.
27. Victora CG, Adair L, Fall C, Hallal PC, Martorell R, Richter L, et al. Maternal and child undernutrition: consequences for adult health and human capital. Lancet. 2008;371(9609):340–57.
28. Lindsay AC, Sussner KM, Kim J, Gortmaker S. The role of parents in preventing childhood obesity. Future Child. 2006;16(1):169–86.
29. Birch LL, Fisher JO. Development of eating behaviors among children and adolescents. Pediatrics. 1998;101(Suppl 2):539–49.
30. Videon TM, Manning CK. Influences on adolescent eating patterns: the importance of family meals. J Adolesc Health. 2003;32(5):365–73.
31. Smith AD, Fildes A, Cooke L, Herle M, Shakeshaft N, Plomin R, et al. Genetic and environmental influences on food preferences in adolescence. Am J Clin Nutr. 2016;104(2):446–53.
32. Salvy S-J, de la Haye K, Bowker JC, Hermans RCJ. Influence of peers and friends on children's and adolescents' eating and activity behaviors. Physiol Behav. 2012;106(3):369–78.
33. Todd AS, Street SJ, Ziviani J, Byrne NM, Hills AP. Overweight and obese adolescent girls: the importance of promoting sensible eating and activity behaviors from the start of the adolescent period. Int J Environ Res Public Health. 2015;12(2):2306–29.
34. Hu T, Jacobs DR Jr, Larson NI, Cutler GJ, Laska MN, Neumark-Sztainer D. Higher diet quality in adolescence and dietary improvements are related to less weight gain during the transition from adolescence to adulthood. J Pediatr. 2016;178:188–93.e3.
35. World Health Organization. Global action plan for the prevention and control of noncommunicable diseases 2013-2020; 2013.
36. United Nations General Assembly. Political declaration of the high-level meeting of the General Assembly on the prevention and control of non-communicable diseases. New York: United Nations; 2011.
37. World Health Organization. Report of the commission on ending childhood obesity. Geneva: World Health Organization; 2016.

38. Khambalia AZ, Dickinson S, Hardy LL, Gill T, Baur LA. A synthesis of existing systematic reviews and meta-analyses of school-based behavioural interventions for controlling and preventing obesity. Obes Rev. 2012;13(3):214–33.
39. Waters E, de Silva-Sanigorski A, Hall BJ, Brown T, Campbell KJ, Gao Y, et al. Interventions for preventing obesity in children. Cochrane Database Syst Rev. 2011;(12):CD001781.
40. Wildridge V, Childs S, Cawthra L, Madge B. How to create successful partnerships—a review of the literature. Health Info Libr J. 2004;21:3–19.
41. Keshavarz Mohammadi N, Rowling L, Nutbeam D. Acknowledging educational perspectives on health promoting schools. Health Educ. 2010;110(4):240–51.
42. Haque B. Changing our secondary schools. Wellington: NZCER Press; 2015.
43. Tucker C, Taylor D. Good science: principles of community-based participatory research. Race Poverty Environ. 2004;11(2):27–9.
44. Rychen DS, Salganik LH, editors. Key competencies for a successful life and well-functioning society. Cambridge: Hogrefe Publishing; 2003.
45. Perkins D. Future wise: educating our children for a changing world. New York: Wiley; 2014.
46. Hipkins R, Bolstad R, Boyd S, McDowall S. Key competencies for the future. Wellington: NZCER Press; 2014.
47. Kahn S, Zeidler DL. Using our heads and HARTSS*: developing perspective-taking skills for socioscientific reasoning (*Humanities, ARTs, and Social Sciences). J Sci Teach Educ. 2016;27(3):261–81.
48. Bronfenbrenner U. Ecological systems theory. Ann Child Dev. 1989;6:187–224.
49. Eidelson RJ. Complex adaptive systems in the behavioral and social sciences. Rev Gen Psychol. 1997;1(1):42–71.
50. Bronfenbrenner U. Making human beings human: bioecological perspectives on human development. Sage: Thousand Oaks; 2005.
51. Endo A, Oyamada M. On Japanese female university students' perception of developmental origins of health and disease: a questionnaire survey. J Dev Orig Health Dis. 2013;4(Suppl 2):S162.
52. Bay J, Dixon R, Morgan S, Wall C, Oyamada M. Characterising public understanding of DOHaD to inform communication strategies. J Dev Orig Health Dis. 2015;6:S2.
53. Bay JL, Mora HA, Sloboda DM, Morton SM, Vickers MH, Gluckman PD. Adolescent understanding of DOHaD concepts: a school-based intervention to support knowledge translation and behaviour change. J Dev Orig Health Dis. 2012;3(6):469–82.
54. Bay JL, Spiroski AM, Fogg-Rogers L, McCann CM, Faull RL, Barber PA. Stroke awareness and knowledge in an urban New Zealand population. J Stroke Cerebrovasc Dis. 2015;24(6):1153–62.
55. Bay JL, Yaqona D, Tairea K, Morgan S, Morgan T, Vickers MH, Barrett-Watson C, Martin J, Herrmann U. The healthy start to life education for adolescents project: indicators of early success in adaptation for use in Small Island Developing States. J Dev Orig Health Dis. 2015;6(S2):S77.
56. Grace M, Woods-Townsend K, Griffiths J, Godfrey K, Hanson M, Galloway I, et al. Developing teenagers' views on their health and the health of their future children. Health Educ. 2012;112(6):543–59.
57. Gage H, Raats M, Williams P, Egan B, Jakobik V, Laitinen K. Developmental origins of health and disease: the views of first-time mothers in 5 European countries on the importance of nutritional influences in the first year of life. Am J Clin Nutr. 2011;94(6 Suppl):2018S–24S.
58. Bay JL, Vickers MH, Mora HA, Sloboda DM, Morton SM. Adolescents as agents of healthful change through scientific literacy development: a school-university partnership program in New Zealand. Int J STEM Educ. 2017;4(1):15. https://doi.org/10.1186/s40594-017-0077-0.
59. Grace M, Bay J. Developing a pedagogy to support science for health literacy. Asia-Pac Forum Sci Learn Teach. 2011;12(2):1–13.
60. Bay JL. My First 1000 Days. Auckland: Read Pacific Publishers Ltd; 2016.
61. Bay JL, Sloboda DM, Vickers MH, Mora HA. Multi-dimensional connections. In: France B, Compton V, editors. Bringing communities together: connecting learners with scientists or technologists. Rotterdam: Sense Publishers; 2012. p. 161–73.

62. New Zealand Ministry of Health. Understanding excess body weight: New Zealand health survey. Wellington: New Zealand Ministry of Health; 2015.
63. Gates MF. Putting women and girls at the center of development. Science. 2014;345(6202):1273–5.
64. Richardson SS, Daniels CR, Gillman MW, Golden J, Kukla R, Kuzawa C, et al. Society: don't blame the mothers. Nature. 2014;512:131–2.
65. Lane M, Zander-Fox DL, Robker RL, McPherson NO. Peri-conception parental obesity, reproductive health, and transgenerational impacts. Trends Endocrinol Metab. 2015;26(2):84–90.
66. Bay JL, Mora HA, Tairea K, Yaqona D, Sloboda DM, Vickers MH. Te maki toto vene (T2): e manamanata no toku iti tangata. Teacher resource. Auckland: Read Pacific Publishers Ltd; 2016.
67. Bay JL, Fehoko F, La'akulu M, Leota O, Pulotu L, Tu'ipoloto S, Tutoe S, Tovo O, Vekoso A, Pouvalu EH. Questioning in Tongan science classrooms: a pilot study to identify current practice, barriers and facilitators. Asia Pac Forum Sci Learn Teach. 2016;17(2):Article 10.
68. Ora TM. Ministry of Health Cook Islands. Cook Islands STEPS survey 2004 vs 2015 fact sheet. Cook Islands Ministry of Health.
69. Neely E, Walton M, Stephens C. Young people's food practices and social relationships. A thematic synthesis. Appetite. 2014;82:50–60. https://doi.org/10.1016/j.appet.2014.07.005.
70. United Nations General Assembly. Universal declaration of human rights: United Nations, 217A, Article 27(i), 1948. www.un.org/en/universal-declaration-human-rights. Accessed 3 Jan 2017.
71. Crosbie J. Ending childhood obesity—a youth perspective: address to the WHA Side Event, Ending Childhood Obesity: securing the future for our children. Sixty-ninth World Health Assembly May 26, 2016; Geneva, Switzerland. http://www.who.int/end-childhood-obesity/news/wha69-event/en/. Accessed 3 Jan 2017.

Chapter 4
Developmental Origins of Health and Disease (DOHaD) Cohorts and Interventions: Status and Perspective

Fumihiro Sata

Abstract The concept of Developmental Origins of Health and Disease (DOHaD), which has emerged over the past decades, links the state of health and disease in later life with environmental factors of the early life. It was the pioneer work of David J. Barker, Southampton University, United Kingdom, who proposed the fetal origins of adult disease hypothesis, also referred to as the "thrifty phenotype" hypothesis or Barker hypothesis, which states that an adverse fetal environmental, such as undernutrition, increases the risk of noncommunicable diseases (NCDs) in adulthood. At the beginning of this century, the DOHaD theory incorporated much broader concepts: not only were poor physical conditions in adulthood, such as disease suffering, strongly associated with the fetal and infant environment, but also the ability to maintain a healthy lifestyle. Currently, the belief that adverse fetal-childhood environments, such as undernutrition, stress, smoking, and chemical exposure due to growth restriction, increases the risk of NCDs in adulthood, such as cardiovascular disease, stroke, hypertension, type 2 diabetes, chronic kidney disease, osteoporosis, cancer, and psychiatric disorders, is widely accepted. In Europe and America, birth cohort studies are very popular because they enable the integration of data sharing and meta-analyses for genome-wide association studies, epigenome-wide association studies, exposome, Mendelian randomization, and early intervention studies. Recently, in Japan, the concept of preemptive medicine, which is a novel medical paradigm that advocates for presymptomatic diagnosis, prediction, or intervention at an early stage to prevent or delay disease onset, has been proposed. Therefore, interdisciplinary studies that focus on fetal and childhood developmental periods are highly recommended as a political strategy. In this chapter, I will introduce DOHaD cohort studies and interventions and discuss their statuses and perspectives.

F. Sata
Health Center, Chuo University, Tokyo, Japan
e-mail: fsata.16h@g.chuo-u.ac.jp

F. Sata et al. (eds.), *Pre-emptive Medicine: Public Health Aspects of Developmental Origins of Health and Disease*, Current Topics in Environmental Health and Preventive Medicine, https://doi.org/10.1007/978-981-13-2194-8_4

Keywords DOHaD · Cohort studies · Interventions · Noncommunicable diseases (NCDs)

Abbreviations

BMI	Body mass index
BW	Birth weight
DOHaD	Developmental Origins of Health and Disease
EWAS	Epigenome-wide association study
GWAS	Genome-wide association study
NCDs	Non-communicable diseases
SNP	Single nucleotide polymorphism

4.1 Introduction

The Developmental Origins of Health and Disease (DOHaD) is a concept that has emerged over the past decades. It links the state of health and disease in later childhood and adult life with environmental factors of the early life, specifically the preconceptional, prenatal, and/or early postnatal periods. It was the pioneer work of David J. Barker, an epidemiologist at Southampton University in the United Kingdom, who conducted a series of descriptive epidemiological studies in England and Wales in the 1980s and found that mortality associated with cardiovascular disease appeared higher in the areas with higher infant mortality rates several decades before. By obtaining data from the Hertfordshire Cohort Study, a prospective survey that recorded all births in Hertfordshire from 1911 until 1948, Barker et al. showed that mortality rates for cardiovascular disease increased in individuals who had lower birth weights and with hypertension and impaired glucose tolerance displaying similar trends [1–4]. Based on these findings, Barker et al. proposed the hypothesis of the fetal origins of adult disease, also referred to as the "thrifty phenotype" hypothesis or the Barker hypothesis, which states that an adverse fetal environmental, such as undernutrition, increases the risk of noncommunicable diseases (NCDs) in adulthood [5–8].

At the beginning of this century, the DOHaD theory incorporated much broader concepts: not only were poor physical conditions in adulthood, such as disease suffering, strongly associated with the fetal environment, but also the ability to maintain a healthy lifestyle [9, 10]. Thus, this theory is a subset of the biological phenomenon of developmental plasticity, which encompasses those processes that generate alternative phenotypes from gene expression through the actions of environmental clues acting during developmental periods. Through the epigenetic control mechanism, also known as developmental programming, the most desirable phenotype is produced in response to the fetal environment to increase the likelihood of postnatal survival [11, 12]. Therefore, if the postnatal environment matches the fetal environment, such as the maintenance of similar nutritional and physical conditions, then the individual will most likely sustain a healthy lifestyle after birth. Conversely, if the postnatal environment does not match the fetal environment, such as poor dietary and physical habits, then the individual will most likely succumb to an unhealthy lifestyle and have a higher risk for NCDs later in life. The DOHaD theory correlates fetal-childhood environmental factors with the incidence of NCDs in adulthood, and this concept has been supported by numerous epidemiological, birth cohort, and experimental studies.

Currently, the belief that adverse fetal-childhood environments, such as undernutrition, stress, smoking, and chemical exposure due to growth restriction, increases the risk of adulthood NCDs, such as cardiovascular disease, stroke, hypertension, type 2 diabetes, chronic kidney disease, osteoporosis, cancer, and psychiatric disorders, is widely accepted.

4.2 Status of Birth Cohort Studies

In Europe and America, birth cohort studies are very popular because they enable the integration of data sharing and meta-analyses (Tables 4.1 and 4.2). Birthcohorts.net, a database of birth cohort networks, has approximately 70 birth cohort studies registered predominantly in Europe that meets the following criteria: initiated in 1980 or later, have at least 300 mother-child pairs, have at least 1 year of follow-up, and provide well-documented data, including questionnaire data and biological samples with appropriate times of collection [13, 14]. The Environmental Health Risks in European Birth Cohorts (ENRIECO) is a project dedicated to environmental risk assessment of chemical substances based on Birthcohorts.net data [15]. The executive committee of the European Union (EU) developed the Child Cohort Research Strategy for Europe (CHICOS) under the 7th Framework Program (7FP) of the European Commission to integrate and evaluate data from existing cohort studies, registration systems, and related European databases to construct health data banks that can be used over the next 15 years [16]. In the United Kingdom, the Cohort and Longitudinal Studies Enhancement Resources (CLOSER) consolidated eight representative birth cohort studies with different starting times to evaluate socioeconomic and biological factors and apply them for health policy [17]. In Asia, the Birth Cohort Consortium of Asia (BiCCA) is a consortium specializing in children's environmental health and is composed of 27 birth cohorts in East Asia, mainly in Japan, China, Korea, and Taiwan [18]. Recently, two birth cohort consortia specializing in genome-wide association studies (GWAS), the Early Growth Genetics (EGG) Consortium and EArly Genetics and Lifecourse Epidemiology (EAGLE) Consortium, have been established [19, 20]. The International Fetal and Newborn Growth Consortium (Intergrowth-21st) is a collaborative research effort on behalf of eight countries, including the United Kingdom, the United States, and China, to evaluate infant growth from the fetal period to early childhood [21]. As more data are collected on the health and nutrition of participating mothers, Intergrowth-21st will use the findings to implement appropriate prenatal care.

Table 4.1 Overview of epidemiological studies associated with Developmental Origins of Health and Disease (DOHaD)

Year	Concept/theory	Descriptive epidemiology	Observational studies	Intervention/proposal
1980		**England and Wales** a strong geographical relation between ischemic heart disease mortality rates and infant mortality several decades ago (Lancet 1986)		
1990	**Barker hypothesis** **Fetal origins of adult disease** (BMJ 1990, Fetal Matern Med Rev 1994, Int J Epidemiol 2002) **Brenner Hypothesis** (Bull Mem Acad R Med Belg 1994)		**Hertfordshire Cohort Study** [***birth weight***] coronary heart disease, hypertension, impaired glucose tolerance (Lancet 1989, BMJ 1991) **Dutch Hunger Winter of 1944–1945** [***prenatal famine***] Schizophrenia (Arch Gen Psychiatry 1992, 1996) **Nurses' Health Study** [***birth weight***] cardiovascular disease (BMJ 1997)	
2000	**Developmental Origins of Health and Disease (DOHaD)** • Mismatch concept • Developmental plasticity (Science 2004; Nature 2004)	**Japan (1980–present)** Increasing prevalence of low birth weight (Lancet 2007, OECD Health Statistics 2016)	**Helsinki Birth Cohort** [***catch-up growth***] coronary heart disease (N Engl J Med 2005) **Chinese famine of 1959–1961** [***prenatal famine***] Schizophrenia (JAMA 2005) **Genome-wide association study (GWAS) – ALSPAC, NFBC1966** [***BMI, obesity***] ***FTO*** (Science 2007)	**Ministry of Health, Labour and Welfare** Dietary Guidelines for Pregnant and Lactating Women (2006) **Science Council of Japan** [Proposal] Prevention against lifestyle-related diseases from prenatal and childhood (2008)

2010			**– EGG/EAGLE Consortium** [***BMI, obesity***] ***OLFM4, HOXB5*** (Nat Genet 2012) [***birth weight***] ***CCNL1, ADCY5, CDKAL1, ADRB1, HMGA2, LCORL, et al.*** (Nat Genet 2010, 2013; Nature 2016) [***birth head circumference***] ***12q15, 12q24, 17q21*** (Nat Genet 2012) [***birth length***] ***DCST2, GDF6, TTC17-HSD17B12, LCORL, PTCH1, GPR126, HMGA2*** (Hum Mol Genet 2015) **Epigenome-wide association study (EWAS)** **– MoBa** [***maternal smoking***] ***AHRR, CYP1A1, GFI1*** (Environ Health Perspect 2012) [***birth weight***] ***ARID5B, XRCC3*** (Am J Epidemiol 2014) **– Dutch** Hunger Winter of 1944–1945 [***birth weight***] ***INSR, CPTA1*** (Nat Commun 2014) **– PACE** [***maternal smoking***] ***AHRR, MYO1G, CNTNAP2, GFI1, et al.*** (Am J Hum Genet 2016) **Mendelian Randomization** **– EGG Consortium** [***birth weight***] Maternal obesity-related traits (JAMA 2016) **Exposome** **– EXPOsOMICS project** (Int J Hyg Environ Health 2016)	**Southampton Women's Survey (SWS): Southampton Initiative for Health** Intervention for disadvantaged women (J Health Psychol 2011; J Dev Orig Health Dis 2016; Healthcare 2017) **EarlyNutrition Project** Randomized controlled trial, e-learning, EarlyNutrition Academy (Proc Nutr Soc 2012; Ann Nutr Metab 2014) **Liggins Education Network for Science (LENScience)** School-based intervention (J Dev Orig Health Dis 2012; Healthcare 2014; Health Promot Int 2017) **Japan Science and Technology Agency (JST)** [Strategic Proposal] Promoting Life Course Healthcare: Importance of Preemptive Medicine in pregnancy to childhood (2014) [Overlooking Report of Research and Development] Life Science and Clinical Research Fields (2015)

[Abbreviations] *ALSPAC* Avon Longitudinal Study of Parents and Children, *NFBC1966* Northern Finland Birth Cohort 1966, *EGG* Early Growth Genetics, *EAGLE* EArly Genetics and Lifecourse Epidemiology, *MoBa* Norwegian Mother and Child Cohort Study, *PACE* Pregnancy And Childhood Epigenetics Consortium

Table 4.2 Major consortia based on birth cohort studies in the world

Consortia	Objective	Participant birth cohorts
CHICOS	– Data sharing – Integrated healthcare database construction	[Belgium] FLEHS, [Czech] Czech Early Childhood Health, [Denmark] ABC, CCC2000, COPSAC-2010, DARC, DNBC, HHf2, IVAAQ, Lupercus, Odense Child Cohort, [Faroe Islands] CHEF, [Finland] LUKAS, NFBC 1986, [France] EDEN, ELFE, PARIS, PÉLAGIE, TIMOUN, [Germany] BabyCare cohort, CHOP, DONALD, Duisburg, GINIplus, LeuBiCo, Life Child, LISA-PLUS, MAS 5, MAS-90, SNiP, [Greece] RHEA, [Ireland] BASELINE, Growing up in Ireland, Lifeways Cross-Generation Cohort Study, [Italy] Co.N.ER, GASPII, MUBICOS, NINFEA, Piccolipiù, Trieste child development cohort, [Lithuania] KANC, [Netherlands] ABCD, GECKO Drenthe cohort, Generation R, KOALA, MEFAB, PIAMA, Predict Study, PRIDE Study, WHISTLER, [Norway] ArcRisk, HUMIS, MoBa, NorFlu, [Poland] Krakow cohort, REPRO_PL, [Portugal] G21, [Slovakia] PCB Cohort, [Spain] INMA Project, [Sweden] ABIS, BAMSE, INUENDO, [Switzerland] BILD, [Ukraine] FCOU, [United Kingdom] ALSPAC, BiB, Determination of maternal caffeine intakes associated with increased risk to the fetus, EHL, GMS, GUS, Isle of Wight Birth Cohort study, LRC, Merthyr Allergy Study, NCCGP, Newcastle Thousand Families Study, SEATON, SWS
CLOSER	– Data harmonization – Data linkage – CLOSER search platform – Research impact – Training and capacity building	HCS, NSHD/1946BC, NCDS, BCS70, ALSPAC, SWS, MCS, UKHLS
ENRIECO	– Environmental health risk assessment	ABC, ABCD, ALSPAC, BAMSE, BiB, CHEF, DBNC, EDEN, ELFE, FLEHS, Generation R, G21, GINIplus, INMA Project, INUENDO, KOALA, LRC, LISA-PLUS, NFBC 1966, NFBC 1986, NINFEA, PIAMA, RHEA, SNiP
BiCCA	– Environmental health risk assessment	[Bangladesh] HRBC, [China] LWBC, NJMUBC, SBC, [Japan] HBC study, Hokkaido Study, TSCD, [Korea] CHECK, COCOA, EDC study, MOCEH, PSKC, [Malaysia] USM pregnancy cohort, [Mongolia] Birth Cohort Study in Mongolia, UGAAR Study, [Nepal] Nepali, [Philippines] CLHNS, [Singapore] GUSTO, [Sri Lanka] KCHS, [Taiwan] TBPS, TEC, TMICS, [United Arab Emirates] MISC, [Vietnam] Bien Hoa study, DaDoCiV, DaNang

Table 4.2 (continued)

Consortia	Objective	Participant birth cohorts
EGG	– GWAS	ALSPAC, CHOP, CoLaus study, COPSAC, DNBC, EFSOCH, ERF, EPIC, Fenland Study, Generation R, GINI-plus, GOYA, HCS, HBCS, INMA Project, Inter99, Leipzig, LISA-plus, NCDS, NEO, NFBC1966, NFBC1986, NTR, ORCADES, PANIC, PIAMA, RAINE, Sorbs, STRIP, TEENAGE, TDCOB, YFS
EAGLE	– GWAS	NCDS, ALSPAC, CATSS, CHOP, COPSAC, DNBC, Exeter Family Study, Generation R, GINI-plus, HBCS, INMA, LISA-plus, MoBa, NTR, NFBC, Project Viva, TCHAD, TEDS, RAINE
Intergrowth-21st	– Scientifically robust clinical tools to assess fetal growth and the nutritional status of newborn infants	Research units in Brazil, China, India, Italy, Kenya, Oman, the United Kingdom, and United States
EpiGen	– EWAS	Liggins Institute, University of Auckland, represented in the consortium by Auckland UniServices Ltd Human Development and Health Academic Unit, University of Southampton MRC Lifecourse Epidemiology Unit, University of Southampton Singapore Institute for Clinical Sciences, Agency for Science, Technology and Research National University of Singapore
PACE	– EWAS	ALSPAC, CHAMACOS, CHS, GECKO Drenthe Cohort, Generation R, IOW, MeDALL, which includes four component cohorts (INMA, EDEN, BAMSE, PIAMA), MoBa, NFCS, NEST, Project Viva, GALA II, SEED
EXPOsOMICS	– Exposome	RHEA, Piccoli+, INMA, ALSPAC

Abbreviations: Appendix B

In addition, worldwide consortia have been developed that specifically address the underlying tenets of the DOHaD theory. Researchers in New Zealand, the United Kingdom, and Singapore are participating in an international consortium, the EpiGen Global Research Consortium, in an effort to use epigenetic techniques and tools for early intervention in at risk pregnant women and children [22, 23]. The Pregnancy And Childhood Epigenetics (PACE) consortium is comprised of researchers at the National Institute of Environmental Health Sciences (NIEHS) and around the world who are using epigenetics to investigate how early-life environmental factors impact human disease [24, 25]. Recently, a need arose for the development of methodology that analyzes an individual's environmental exposure with the same precision of GWAS or whole genome sequencing methods. Christopher P. Wild, Chair of Molecular Epidemiology at the University of Leeds and Director of the International Agency for Research on Cancer (IARC), proposed the need for an "exposome" to match the "genome," to raise awareness for exposure assessment methodology [26]. An EU-funded project, EXPOsOMICS, aims to develop a novel approach for assessing exposure to high-priority environmental pollutants, such as air and water contaminants, during critical periods of life by characterizing the external and internal components of the exposome [27]. Yet, Mendelian randomization is a GWAS-based theoretical method for environmental risk assessment that uses genetic factors associated with environmental factors to assess the causal effect on internal biomarkers, such as body mass index (BMI), systolic blood pressure, and fasting glucose levels [28].

4.3 Genome-Wide Epidemiological Researches in Birth Cohorts

In adult cohort studies, GWAS have aided in the development of the DNA microarray technique and have been actively performed to elucidate associations between various outcomes such as traits and diseases and genetic factors, with numerous genome cohorts establishing specific consortia to perform data integration and meta-analysis for each outcome. In 2007, *Science* magazine named "human genetic variation" as the breakthrough of the year because of the tremendous advancement in the understanding of how genomes differ from one human to another [29]. Since then, GWAS reports have dramatically increased [30, 31], and several consortia specializing in GWAS meta-analyses of birth cohort studies, such as the EGG and EAGLE Consortia, have been established [19, 20]. These consortia have conducted risk evaluation of various outcomes from the viewpoint of life-course epidemiology, and in cooperation with consortia that have already been established in adult cohort studies, these consortia have contributed to the identification of associations between childhood factors and adulthood NCDs or traits that developed over time [32–36].

Since GWAS have been conducted in adult genome cohort studies, a small number of birth cohort studies have also participated in GWAS. Of particular prominence, in one of these studies, an association of a single nucleotide polymorphism (SNP) rs9939609 in the obesity-associated *FTO* gene with BMI, obesity risk, and type 2 diabetes was detected in multiple populations [32]. The association between BMI and this SNP has been confirmed in a total of 38,759 participants from 13 cohort studies, including two birth cohort studies: the Avon Longitudinal Study of Parents and Children (ALSPAC) and the Northern Finland Birth Cohort 1966 (NFBC 1966), which participated in the EGG and EAGLE Consortia. The 16% of adults who were homozygous for the risk allele weighed approximately 3 kg more than adults who did not inherit the risk allele and had 1.67-fold increase in odds for obesity; this observation was seen in subjects over the age of 7 years and reflected a specific increase in fat mass [32]. Regarding early-onset obesity, meta-analysis was conducted for the 13,848 participants of European descent from 14 cohort studies in North America, Europe, and Australia, who were also included in the EGG Consortium (5530 obese people with a BMI greater than the 95th percentile and 8318 controls with a BMI less than the 50th percentile) [33]. According to this large-scale study, two genetic loci, rs9568856 near the *OLFM4* gene and rs9299 of the *HOXB5* gene, were detected at the genome-wide significance level. Meta-analysis also revealed a significant association between these loci and adult BMI.

In addition, the EGG Consortium conducted a GWAS of the 10,623 participants of European descent from 13 birth cohorts and found that two genetic loci, rs900400 near the *CCNL1* gene and rs9883204 in the *ADCY5* gene, were significantly associated with birth weight (BW) regarded as indicators of fetal growth [34]. Correlated SNPs in the *ADCY5* gene were implicated in the regulation of glucose levels and increased susceptibility to type 2 diabetes, providing evidence that the well-described association between lower birth weight and subsequent type 2 diabetes has a genetic component, which is distinct from the proposed role of programming by maternal nutrition [34]. However, since this SNP has not been detected in individuals of Japanese descent, the marker cannot be used to evaluate Japanese populations. Next, the EGG and EAGLE Consortia conducted an expanded genome-wide association meta-analysis and follow-up study of BW for 69,308 individuals of European descent from 43 studies [35]. This large-scale study increased the number of loci detected at the genome-wide significance level to seven (*CCNL1*, *ADCY5*, *HMGA2*, *CDKAL1*, *5q11.2*, *LCORL*, and *ADRB1*), accounting for a variance proportion similar to that of maternal smoking. Five of the loci are known to be associated with other phenotypes: *ADCY5* and *CDKAL1* with type 2 diabetes, *ADRB1* with adult blood pressure, and *HMGA2* and *LCORL* with adult height [35]. These findings highlight genetic links between fetal growth, postnatal growth, and metabolism. Recently, the EGG and EAGLE Consortia performed a multi-ancestry GWAS meta-analysis of BW in 153,781 individuals participating in the EGG Consortium or UK Biobank and identified 60 loci where the fetal genotype was associated with BW [36]. Genetic correlations between BW and other health-related traits were estimated using linkage-disequilibrium score regression, which showed that BW had a strong positive genetic correlation with anthropometric and obesity-related traits, including birth length and, in adults, height, waist circumference, and BMI, while BW had an inverse genetic correlation with indicators of adverse metabolic and cardiovascular health, including coronary artery disease, systolic blood pressure, and type 2 diabetes (Figs. 4.1 and 4.2). For example, BW-associated regions, such as *CDKAL1*, *HHEX-IDE*, *MTNR1B*, *PLEKHA1*, *ADCY5*, and *ANK1*, are associated with type 2 diabetes, while *NT5C2*, *FES*, *EBF1*, *NRIP1*, and *ADRB1* are associated with systolic blood pressure, and *NT5C2* and *LCORL* are associated with coronary artery disease. Thus, big data from large-scale genome cohort studies suggest that life-course associations between early growth phenotypes and adult NCDs and traits may be genetically linked.

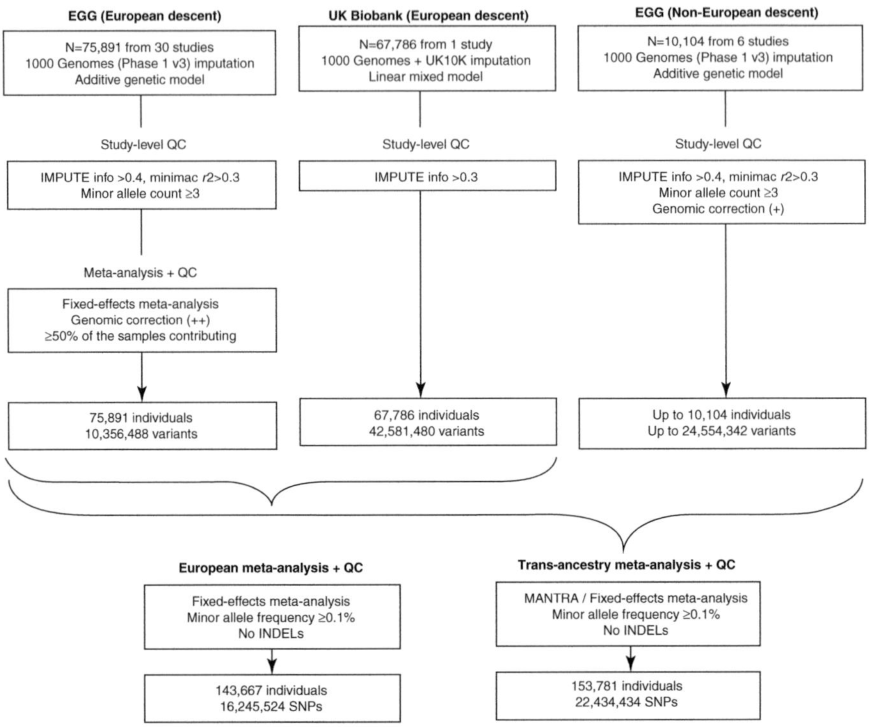

Fig. 4.1 Flow chart of the study design [36]

4.4 Birth Cohort-Based Evaluation of Epigenetic Changes and Exposome Reflecting Long-Term Environmental Exposures

Epigenetics refers to DNA modifications that do not alter the DNA sequence but instead reflect intergenerational environmental effects. In consideration of the DOHaD theory, epigenetic modifications, such as DNA methylation, caused by in utero exposures may play a critical role in early programming for the development of childhood and adult diseases. Epigenome-wide association studies (EWAS) have been employed to detect whole genome DNA methylation. Maternal smoking during pregnancy is a major risk factor for multiple adverse health outcomes in children, but the underlying mechanisms remain unclear. Norwegian researchers measured maternal plasma cotinine, an objective biomarker of smoking, during pregnancy in relation to DNA methylation at 473,844 CpG sites (CpGs) in 1062 newborn cord blood samples from the Norwegian Mother and Child Cohort Study (MoBa). Differential DNA methylation at epigenome-wide statistical significance was found for 26 CpGs mapped to 10 genes, and a US birth cohort study replicated the findings for CpGs in *AHRR*, *CYP1A1*, and *GFI1* at multiple comparison statistical significance [37]. Of the detected genes,

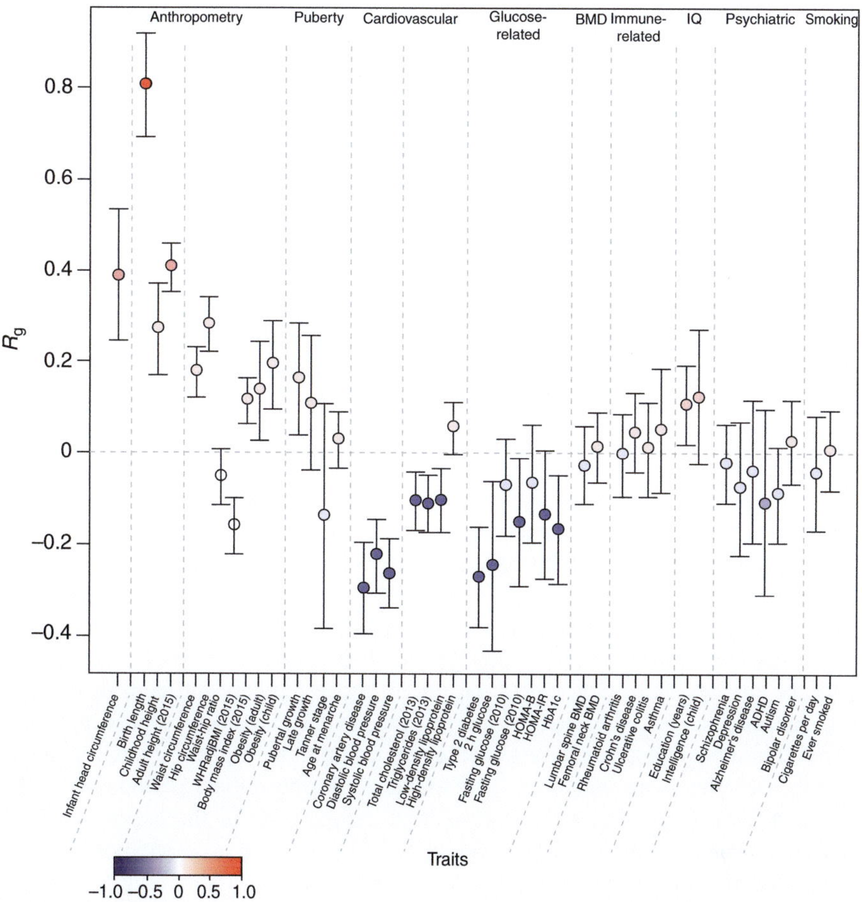

Fig. 4.2 Genome-wide genetic correlation between BW and a range of traits and diseases in later life [36]. Genetic correlation (R_g) and corresponding s.e. (error bars) between BW and the traits displayed on the *x* axis were estimated using linkage-disequilibrium score regression. The genetic correlation estimates (R_g) are color coded according to their intensity and direction (red for positive and blue for inverse correlation). *WHRadjBMI* waist-hip ratio adjusted for body mass index, *HOMA-B/IR* homeostasis model assessment of beta-cell function/insulin resistance, *HbA1c* hemoglobin A1c, *BMD* bone mineral density, *ADHD* attention deficit hyperactivity disorder

AHRR and *CYP1A1* play a key role in the aryl hydrocarbon receptor signaling pathway, which mediates the detoxification of smoking residuals. Recently, the PACE consortium completed a meta-analysis across 13 cohorts ($n = 6685$) and found cohort-specific associations between maternal smoking during pregnancy and DNA methylation in the offspring [25]. DNA methylation was detected at over 450,000 CpGs, and over 6000 of these CpGs, including CpGs in *AHRR*, *CYP1A1*, *GFI1*, *MYO1G*, and *CNTNAP2*, were differentially methylated in relation to maternal smoking at the genome-wide statistical significance level [25]. This large-scale meta-analysis of methylation data identified numerous loci involved in response to maternal smoking during pregnancy that persisted into later childhood, thus providing insights into the underlying mechanisms of prenatal effects on later health statuses.

However, environmental exposures that disturb cellular and physiological processes and influence individual predisposition to diseases are likely to do so through active, or reactive, modulation of genome function, through changes in DNA methylation and transcription [38]. The exposome encompasses life-course environmental exposures, including lifestyle factors, from the prenatal period onward. Developing reliable measurement tools for such a complete exposure history is extremely challenging; yet, unlike the genome, the exposome is a highly variable and dynamic entity that evolves throughout an individual's life [26]. To develop a more cohesive view of environmental exposure, recognition must be given to toxic effects mediated through chemicals that alter critical molecules, cells, and physiological processes inside the body [39]. Thus, the environment can be reasonably considered to be the body's internal chemical environment, while exposures can be considered to be the amount of biologically active chemicals found in this internal environment [39]. Through this viewpoint, exposures are not restricted to chemicals entering the body via the air, water, or food but also include chemicals produced by inflammation, oxidative stress, lipid peroxidation, infections, gut flora, and other natural bodily processes. More than a decade has passed since the exposome concept was first proposed, and the subsequent years have been filled with discussions of definitions and challenges of the widespread implementation of the concept into research. However, it is time to move the concept from theory into practice, such as with the establishment of the EXPOsOMICS project, which aims to develop a novel approach for assessing exposure to high-priority environmental pollutants, such as air and water contaminants, during critical periods of life by characterizing the external and the internal components of the exposome [27]. Thus, the project focuses on the following two objectives: to assess exposure at the personal and population level within existing European short- and long-term population studies by exploiting available tools and methods for personal exposure monitoring and to employ multi-omics technologies for the analysis of biological samples, which serve as internal markers of external exposures (Fig. 4.3) [27].

4.5 Prevention of NCDs Through Effective Early Intervention

The first 1000 days of life, spanning from the fetus to the age of 2 years, represents a vulnerable period for programming NCD risk and is an important target for NCD prevention [40, 41]. Successful intervention during this period seems to greatly reduce the risk of NCD development later in life (Fig. 4.4) [42]. In Europe and the United States, a large-scale international collaborative research group has launched a project entitled, "Long-term effects of early nutrition on later health (EarlyNutrition)," to determine the most effective time and method of intervention with the assumption that nutritional intervention during the developmental period reduces the risk of NCDs in both pregnant women and their offspring [43, 44].

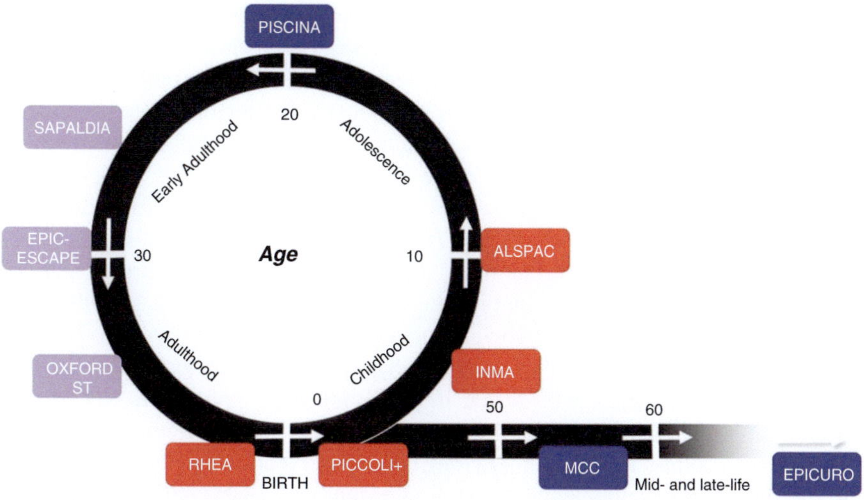

Fig. 4.3 The conceptual framework of EXPOsOMICS (life-long integration of cohorts) [27]

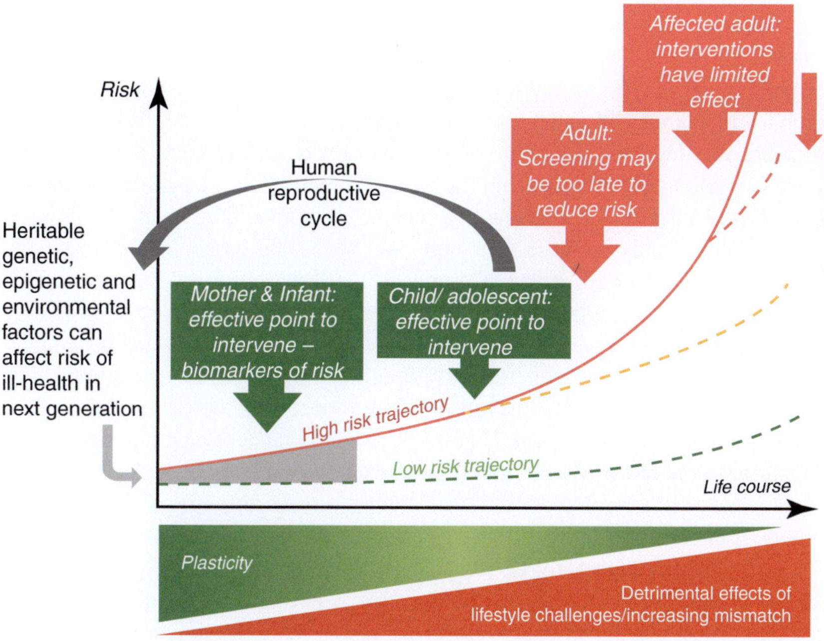

Fig. 4.4 Life-course view of noncommunicable disease (NCD) risk [42]. Risk increases in a nonlinear way as a result of declining plasticity and accumulative damage from lifestyle-imposed or other challenges. The effect of mismatch between developmentally and evolutionarily influenced phenotype and adult environment also increases through the lifecourse. Interventions in adults, especially those at high risk, can be beneficial but only to a degree. Screening in middle-aged adults may also be too late to reduce risk substantially. Interventions in adolescents and young adults are likely to be more effective and, importantly, can reduce the risk of NCDs in the next generation. The prenatal period establishes risk through interaction between genetic, epigenetic, and environmental factors

Using existing cohort studies, ongoing and novel intervention studies, and a basic science program to investigate those key hypotheses, EarlyNutrition will provide the scientific foundations for evidence-based recommendations for optimal nutrition that considers long-term health outcomes, specifically obesity and related disorders. Already, EarlyNutrition has conducted randomized controlled trials for children and has provided educational training for researchers and healthcare professionals. Infant nutrition has a major impact on immediate outcomes, long-term health, and later disease risks, such as obesity and related disorders, and this phenomenon is referred to as "metabolic programming." Rapid weight gain in the first 2 years of life, most notably mediated by dairy protein, affects the insulin-like growth factor metabolic pathways, where epigenetic processes seem to play a role [45]. In addition, the Southampton Women's Survey (SWS), a prospective cohort study targeting women before pregnancy who reside in disadvantaged communities, found that developing sustainable, workable interventions and effective community partnerships requires commitment beginning long before intervention delivery and is key to the translation of developmental research into improved health outcomes [46–48]. On the other hand, Liggins Laboratories in New Zealand launched nutrition educational programs for school children that deploys texts, such as the Liggins Education Network for Science (LENScience), e-learning platforms, and original school-based edible education [49–51]. These programs should be multidisciplinary, utilizing both educational and health expertise, because even though health outcomes may not be evident in the short term, they may occur with learning-related behavior modifications, which are highly effective when sustained over a lifetime [51].

In 2006, the Japanese Ministry of Health, Labor, and Welfare published the "Dietary Guidelines for Pregnant and Lactating Women" [52]. The guideline offered evidence-based information on how pregnant women should consume foods on a daily basis and steadily increase their body weight during pregnancy. However, in 2008, the Science Council of Japan proposed the "prevention of lifestyle-related diseases from prenatal and childhood," which recognized the importance of early intervention [53]. Recently, the concept of preemptive medicine, which is a novel medical paradigm that advocates for presymptomatic diagnosis or prevention intervention at an early stage to prevent disease onset, has been proposed [12]. Traditionally, epidemiological studies often target middle-aged and elderly people, producing an abundance of epidemiological data for subjects over the age of 55 years; however, epidemiological data for subjects under the age of 40 years are extremely limited [54]. Further, biological samples taken from middle-aged or elderly subjects will inherently be affected by the processes of aging, even if the individual is healthy. Therefore, this data source is not suitable for detecting early biomarkers. Thus, current research efforts are recognizing the importance of interdisciplinary research that focuses on the fetal period through childhood, conducts science and technology workshops, and proposes strategic policies that address these issues [55–57]. Research themes that need to be addressed and promoted in the future are classified into three categories (Table 4.3) [56]. Among them, specification of core institutions and organizations that supervise the whole project from a mid- to long-term viewpoint and acquisition of human resources and development of the next generation are important and fundamental items common to all three themes.

Table 4.3 Important themes that should be promoted in the future

Important items common to all three themes
1. Specification of core institutions and organizations that supervise the whole project from a mid- to long-term viewpoint 2. Acquisition of human resources and development of the next generation 3. Appropriate activities in the perspective of ethical, legal, and social implications (ELSI)
Theme 1: Establishment, operation, and utilization of epidemiological bases
1. Integration of existing birth cohorts and biobanks together with formation of consortia 2. Establishment of an environment that facilitates access to the data by researchers 3. Initiation of a new epidemiological foundation that cannot be obtained by existing epidemiological research infrastructure 4. Establishment of new epidemiological bases shall be planned based on thorough discussions including measures to ensure mid- to long-term funding
Theme 2: Promotion of basic and fundamental life science studies
1. Promotion of researches in genome, epigenome, nutrition, disease, and behavioral sciences 2. Promotion of measurement techniques
Theme 3: Promotion of research and development toward social implementation and impact assessment involved with implementation
1. Collecting, managing, and analyzing in detail the big data obtained through promotion of epidemiological studies and life science studies 2. Quantitative assessment of impact on health, economy, and society

4.6 Conclusion

At the beginning of this century, the DOHaD theory incorporated much broader concepts: not only were poor physical conditions in adulthood, such as disease suffering, strongly associated with the fetal environment but also the ability to maintain a healthy lifestyle. Today, adverse fetal-childhood environments, such as undernutrition, stress, smoking, and chemical exposure due to growth restriction, are known to increase the risk of NCDs, such as cardiovascular disease, stroke, hypertension, type 2 diabetes, chronic kidney disease, osteoporosis, cancer, and psychiatric disorders, later in life. Currently, birth cohort studies are establishing consortia together to promote integrated data sharing and meta-analyses for GWAS, EWAS, exposome, Mendelian randomization, and early intervention studies. Recently, in Japan, a new medical paradigm of preemptive medicine was proposed, and policies have been created that emphasize the importance of fetal-childhood research. In particular, I hope Japan as a nation plans and initiates interdisciplinary national-scale, preemptive medicine projects based on the DOHaD theory, establishes a central research institution, and engages in international consortia focused on improving life-course healthcare. I have great expectations for this nation, and I look forward to the future implementation of these initiatives.

References

1. Barker DJ, Osmond C. Infant mortality, childhood nutrition, and ischaemic heart disease in England and Wales. Lancet. 1986;1:1077–81.

2. Barker DJ, Winter PD, Osmond C, Margetts B, Simmonds SJ. Weight in infancy and death from ischaemic heart disease. Lancet. 1989;2:577–80.
3. Hales CN, Barker DJ, Clark PM, Cox LJ, Fall C, Osmond C, et al. Fetal and infant growth and impaired glucose tolerance at age 64. Br Med J. 1991;303:1019–22.
4. Barker DJ, Gluckman PD, Godfrey KM, Harding JE, Owens JA, Robinson JS. Fetal nutrition and cardiovascular disease in adult life. Lancet. 1993;341:938–41.
5. Barker DJ. The fetal and infant origins of adult disease. Br Med J. 1990;301:1111.
6. Barker DJ. The fetal origins of adult disease. Fetal Maternal Med Rev. 1994;6:71–80.
7. Harding JE. The nutritional basis of the fetal origins of adult disease. Int J Epidemiol. 2001;30:15–23.
8. Barker DJ. The fetal origins of adult disease. In: Foyle G & Nathanson V (Eds). Growing Up in the UK: ensuring a healthy future for our children. BMA Science & Education Dept and the Board of Science; 2013. p. 149–68.
9. Gluckman PD, Hanson MA. Living with the past: evolution, development, and patterns of disease. Science. 2004;305:1733–6.
10. Bateson P, Barker D, Clutton-Brock T, Deb D, D'Udine B, Foley RA, et al. Developmental plasticity and human health. Nature. 2004;430:419–21.
11. Godfrey KM, Lillycrop KA, Burdge GC, Gluckman PD, Hanson MA. Epigenetic mechanisms and the mismatch concept of the developmental origins of health and disease. Pediatr Res. 2007;61:5R–10R.
12. Imura H. Life course health care and preemptive approach to non-communicable diseases. Proc Jpn Acad Ser B Phys Biol Sci. 2013;89:462–73.
13. Larsen PS, Kamper-Jørgensen M, Adamson A, Barros H, Bonde JP, Brescianini S, et al. Pregnancy and birth cohort resources in Europe: a large opportunity for aetiological child health research. Paediatr Perinat Epidemiol. 2013;27:393–414.
14. http://www.birthcohorts.net/. Accessed 31 May 2018.
15. http://www.enrieco.org/. Accessed 31 May 2018.
16. http://www.chicosproject.eu/the-project/. Accessed 31 May 2018.
17. http://www.closer.ac.uk/. Accessed 31 May 2018.
18. http://www.bicca.org/. Accessed 31 May 2018.
19. http://egg-consortium.org/. Accessed 31 May 2018.
20. https://www.wikigenes.org/e/art/e/348.html. Accessed 31 May 2018.
21. http://www.intergrowth21.org.uk/. Accessed 31 May 2018.
22. http://www.epigengrc.com/. Accessed 31 May 2018.
23. Lillycrop KA, Costello PM, Teh AL, Murray RJ, Clarke-Harris R, Barton SJ, et al. Association between perinatal methylation of the neuronal differentiation regulator HES1 and later childhood neurocognitive function and behaviour. Int J Epidemiol. 2015;44:1263–76.
24. https://www.niehs.nih.gov/research/atniehs/labs/epi/pi/genetics/pace/index.cfm Accessed 31 May 2018.
25. Joubert BR, Felix JF, Yousefi P, Bakulski KM, Just AC, Breton C, et al. DNA methylation in newborns and maternal smoking in pregnancy: genome-wide consortium meta-analysis. Am J Hum Genet. 2016;98:680–96.
26. Wild CP. Complementing the genome with an "exposome": the outstanding challenge of environmental exposure measurement in molecular epidemiology. Cancer Epidemiol Biomarkers Prev. 2005;14:1847–50.
27. Vineis P, Chadeau-Hyam M, Gmuender H, Gulliver J, Herceg Z, Kleinjans J, et al. The exposome in practice: design of the EXPOsOMICS project. Int J Hyg Environ Health. 2017;220(2 Pt A):142–51.
28. Tyrrell J, Richmond RC, Palmer TM, Feenstra B, Rangarajan J, Metrustry S, et al. Genetic evidence for causal relationships between maternal obesity-related traits and birth weight. JAMA. 2016;315:1129–40.
29. Pennisi E. Breakthrough of the year. Human genetic variation. Science. 2007;318:1842–3.
30. Welter D, MacArthur J, Morales J, Burdett T, Hall P, Junkins H, et al. The NHGRI GWAS Catalog, a curated resource of SNP-trait associations. Nucleic Acids Res. 2014;42:D1001–6.

31. MacArthur J, Bowler E, Cerezo M, Gil L, Hall P, Hastings E, et al. The new NHGRI-EBI Catalog of published genome-wide association studies (GWAS Catalog). Nucleic Acids Res. 2017;45:D896–901.
32. Frayling TM, Timpson NJ, Weedon MN, Zeggini E, Freathy RM, Lindgren CM, et al. A common variant in the FTO gene is associated with body mass index and predisposes to childhood and adult obesity. Science. 2007;316:889–94.
33. Bradfield JP, Taal HR, Timpson NJ, Scherag A, Lecoeur C, Warrington NM, et al. A genome-wide association meta-analysis identifies new childhood obesity loci. Nat Genet. 2012;44:526–31.
34. Freathy RM, Mook-Kanamori DO, Sovio U, Prokopenko I, Timpson NJ, Berry DJ, et al. Variants in ADCY5 and near CCNL1 are associated with fetal growth and birth weight. Nat Genet. 2010;42:430–5.
35. Horikoshi M, Yaghootkar H, Mook-Kanamori DO, Sovio U, Taal HR, Hennig BJ, et al. New loci associated with birth weight identify genetic links between intrauterine growth and adult height and metabolism. Nat Genet. 2013;45:76–82.
36. Horikoshi M, Beaumont RN, Day FR, Warrington NM, Kooijman MN, Fernandez-Tajes J, et al. Genome-wide associations for birth weight and correlations with adult disease. Nature. 2016;538:248–52.
37. Joubert BR, Håberg SE, Nilsen RM, Wang X, Vollset SE, Murphy SK, et al. 450K epigenome-wide scan identifies differential DNA methylation in newborns related to maternal smoking during pregnancy. Environ Health Perspect. 2012;120:1425–31.
38. Franks PW, McCarthy MI. Exposing the exposures responsible for type 2 diabetes and obesity. Science. 2016;354:69–73.
39. Rappaport SM, Smith MT. Epidemiology. Environment and disease risks. Science. 2010;330:460–1.
40. Adair LS. Long-term consequences of nutrition and growth in early childhood and possible preventive interventions. Nestle Nutr Inst Workshop Ser. 2014;78:111–20.
41. Garmendia ML, Corvalan C, Uauy R. Assessing the public health impact of developmental origins of health and disease (DOHaD) nutrition interventions. Ann Nutr Metab. 2014;64:226–30.
42. Hanson MA, Gluckman PD. Early developmental conditioning of later health and disease: physiology or pathophysiology? Physiol Rev. 2014;94:1027–76.
43. Koletzko B, Brands B, Poston L, Godfrey K, Demmelmair H, Early Nutrition Project. Early nutrition programming of long-term health. Proc Nutr Soc. 2012;71:371–8.
44. http://www.project-earlynutrition.eu/index.html. Accessed 31 May 2018.
45. Brands B, Demmelmair H, Koletzko B, EarlyNutrition Project. How growth due to infant nutrition influences obesity and later disease risk. Acta Paediatr. 2014;103:578–85.
46. Barker M, Baird J, Lawrence W, Jarman M, Black C, Barnard K, et al. The Southampton Initiative for Health: a complex intervention to improve the diets and increase the physical activity levels of women from disadvantaged communities. J Health Psychol. 2011;16: 178–91.
47. https://www.mrc.ac.uk/research/facilities-and-resources-for-researchers/cohort-directory/southampton-women-s-survey/. Accessed 31 May 2018.
48. Barker M, Baird J, Tinati T, Vogel C, Strömmer S, Rose T, et al. Translating developmental origins: improving the health of women and their children using a sustainable approach to behaviour change. Healthcare. 2017;5:17.
49. http://www.lenscience.auckland.ac.nz/en.html. Accessed 31 May 2018.
50. Bay JL, Mora HA, Sloboda DM, Morton SM, Vickers MH, Gluckman PD. Adolescent understanding of DOHaD concepts: a school-based intervention to support knowledge translation and behaviour change. J Dev Orig Health Dis. 2012;3:469–82.
51. Bay JL, Hipkins R, Siddiqi K, Huque R, Dixon R, Shirley D, et al. School-based primary NCD risk reduction: education and public health perspectives. Health Promot Int. 2017;32:369–79.
52. Healthy Parents and Children 21 Investigation Committee. Dietary guidelines for pregnant and lactating women. Tokyo: Ministry of Health, Labour, and Welfare; 2006. http://rhino.med.yamanashi.ac.jp/sukoyaka/ninpu_syoku.html. Accessed 31 May 2018 [Japanese].

53. Science Council of Japan. Prevention of life-style-related diseases from prenatal and childhood; 2008.
54. Collins FS, Manolio TA. Merging and emerging cohorts: necessary but not sufficient. Nature. 2007;445:259.
55. Life Science and Clinical Research Unit. Future strategy of science and technology workshop report: refinement of preemptive medical focusing on fetal period to infancy (including childhood). Tokyo: Center for Research and Development Strategy, Japan Science and Technology Agency, 2014.
56. Life Science and Clinical Research Unit. Strategic proposal: proposal for issue-driven research and development III, promoting life course health-care: importance of preemptive medicine in pregnancy to childhood. Tokyo: Center for Research and Development Strategy, Japan Science and Technology Agency; 2014.
57. Life Science and Clinical Research Unit. Overlooking Report of Research and Development: Life Science and clinical Research Fields (2015). Tokyo: Center for Research and Development Strategy, Japan Science and Technology Agency; 2015.

Chapter 5
Science, Technology, and Innovation Policy: Proposal of Preemptive/Precision Medicine Strategy (Including DOHaD)

Masahiro Tsuji

Abstract Prevention is an extremely important part of welfare efforts for humans. I introduce the new concepts of "preemptive medicine" which indicate the direction we should take to realize prevention. As one of the specific R&D strategies toward the realization of prevention, I propose research subjects and a promoting system with a focus on "preemptive medicine/precision medicine (including DOHaD)." Additionally, I propose the measures for promoting the social implementation of technologies for "life-course health care" as a future vision beyond them.

Keywords DOHaD · IoBMT · Life-course health care · Preemptive medicine · Precision medicine · R&D strategy

Abbreviations

DOHaD	Developmental Origins of Health and Disease
IoBMT	Integration of Bio-Medical Things
QALY	Quality-adjusted life year
QOL	Quality of life
R&D	Research and development

M. Tsuji
Life Science and Clinical Research Unit, Center for Research and Development Strategy (CRDS), Japan Science and Technology Agency (JST), Tokyo, Japan
e-mail: tsuji@jst.go.jp

F. Sata et al. (eds.), *Pre-emptive Medicine: Public Health Aspects of Developmental Origins of Health and Disease*, Current Topics in Environmental Health and Preventive Medicine, https://doi.org/10.1007/978-981-13-2194-8_5

5.1 R&D Concept Based on Social Trends in Japan: "Preemptive/Precision Medicine (Including DOHaD)"

5.1.1 Data on Social Trends in Japan

In Japan, the birthrate is decreasing, and the population is aging more rapidly than anywhere else in the world. The total population is expected to decline considerably in the future, and the decline is forecast to be most remarkable in the "working-age population (population 15 to 64 years old)." It is forecast that a "piggyback-like" society where one aged person (65 years old or older) is supported by about 1.3 "working-age persons." Moreover, soaring medical expenses and care expenditure are expected due to advanced medical technologies and increase in medicine/care needs, etc.

These issues are now becoming more and more serious. If this situation is overlooked, we will face a severe and difficult future plagued with declining economic growth caused by reduced domestic demand, declining domestic production capacity caused by the decreased labor force population, the downfall of the medical/care systems, etc. However, this future outlook can be changed by promoting strategic science and technology policies from the medium- and long-term viewpoint as soon as possible.

5.1.2 Viewpoint of the Formulation of an R&D Strategy (Relation with Social Needs)

On the basis of the data on social trends as shown in Table 5.1, the various issues and social needs in Japan may, I believe, be summarized into the following three points.

1. "People" (e.g., many children grow up healthy. Many aged persons have attained a high QOL.)
2. "Government" (e.g., appropriate medical/care systems responding to soaring medical expenses and care expenditure and medical security)
3. "Academia and industry" (e.g., development of science and technology and health care and medical technology and industry activation).

These are all important social needs. However, some parts of them are inconsistent with each other. For example, the needs of the "people" to use the latest medical technologies (extremely high priced in many cases) are inconsistent with the needs of the "government" to control the rapid increase in medical expenses from the standpoint of sustainability of the national finances.

It will be essential for the future policy of science and technology to satisfy social needs from these three points of view "in a well-balanced and simultaneous manner." With a view of realizing such a goal, I have been involved in the collection of information as seen from a bird's-eye view (trends in R&D, science and technology policies, and industries) and discuss R&D strategies with researchers and

Table 5.1 Data of Japan's social trends

	Past	2010	Future forecast
Total population	93 million people (1960)	128 million people (2010)	87 million people (2060)
Working-age population (15–64 years old)	60 million people (1960)	82 million people (2010)	44 million people (2060)
Aging rate (share of the aged population (65 years old or older))	5.7% (1960)	23.0% (2010)	39.9% (2060)
Working-age population supporting an aged person	11 persons (1960)	2.8 persons (2010)	1.3 persons (2060)
Medical expenses	31 trillion yen (2000)	37.8 trillion yen (2010)	54 trillion yen (2025)
Care expenditure	3.6 trillion yen (2000)	8.4 trillion yen (2010)	19.8 trillion yen (2025)
Import surplus (pharmaceuticals)	0.6 billion (2000)	1.9 trillion yen (2014)	–

(Reference: website of the Cabinet Office, the Ministry of Health, Labour and Welfare etc.) [1]

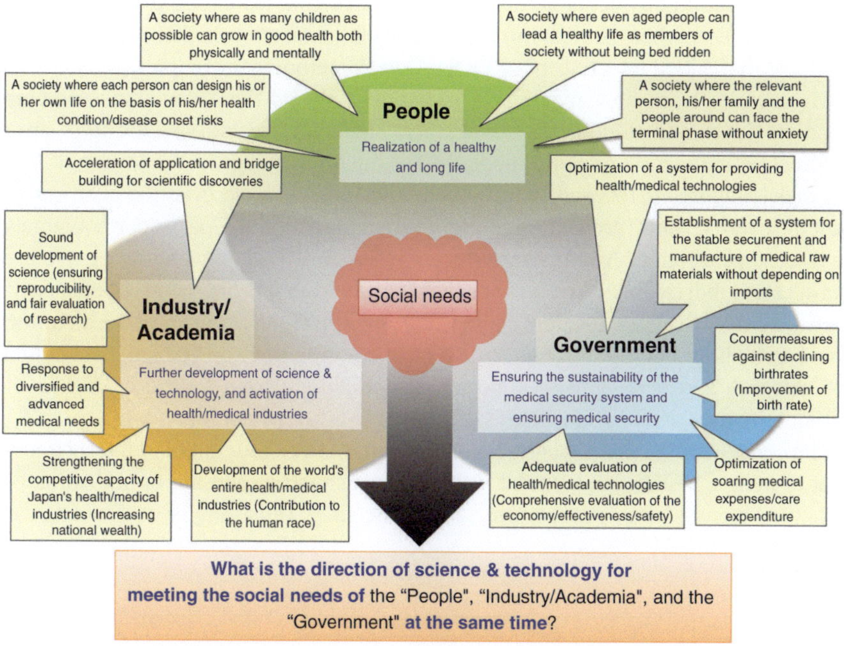

Fig. 5.1 Points of view required for the formulation of R&D strategies Japan ought to pursue (personal views)

policy-making authorities and group workshop. In addition, I support the formulation of specific R&D strategies as well as the initiation of national projects based on the strategies (Fig. 5.1).

5.1.3 New Concepts of Science and Technology: "Preemptive Medicine" and "Precision Medicine"

Diseases expected to decrease the QOL of people and impose a considerable burden on society in the future include cardio-metabolic diseases, chronic obstructive pulmonary disease (COPD), mental disease, dementia, cancer, etc. It is a serious challenge not only for Japan but also for the entire world on how to address these diseases [2].

These diseases are caused by the interaction between genetic predisposition and environmental factors (lifestyles (meals, physical exercise, etc.)) in the long term, coupled with disease risk factors that gradually accumulate and lead to a disease onset. It is not easy to provide curative treatment after the disease onset, and a higher improving effect may be obtained through intervention at an earlier stage. For this reason, in 2010, I proposed a concept of comprehensive disease prevention called "preemptive medicine" [3]. The concept of "preemptive medicine" aims to maintain the health of the people by making use of highly cost-effective intervention technologies (lifestyles (meals, physical exercise, etc.), pharmaceuticals, and so on) and to prevent the disease onset and advancement in severity after identifying high risks by low-cost and highly accurate disease onset prediction technologies (genetic predisposition, biomarker, clinical information, social data, etc.). In 2014 we proposed a concept that added the concept of DOHaD to "preemptive medicine."

Meanwhile, I am now making an in-depth study on the "Precision Medicine Initiative (US)" and re-defining "preemptive medicine (including DOHaD)" in a constructive manner. "Precision medicine (in Japan)" positions, in addition to disease onset prevention, focused on by "preemptive medicine," "prevention of advancement in severity," and "prevention of paroxysm and recurrence" as important targets for disease prevention. And in these three phases of disease prevention, people are stratified and individualized on an appropriate scale from the viewpoints of economy, safety, and effectiveness. In addition, in R&D activities for this purpose, the direction of research should be focused on "IoBMT (Integration of Bio-Medical Things, the new research and development concept we defined)," driven by the collection of high-quality data and big data analyses (including artificial intelligence).

The concept of "preemptive/precision medicine" allows for not only the enhancement of people's QOL but also the activation of industries and the optimization of medical expenses/care expenditure, simultaneously satisfying social needs, as shown in Fig. 5.2.

5.1.4 Materialization of the Concept of "Preemptive/Precision Medicine"

Both a technology to "forecast" the onset/advancement in severity/paroxysm and recurrence of a disease and a technology to "intervention" in curative measures are needed to realize "preemptive/precision medicine." The overview of these technologies is as follows:

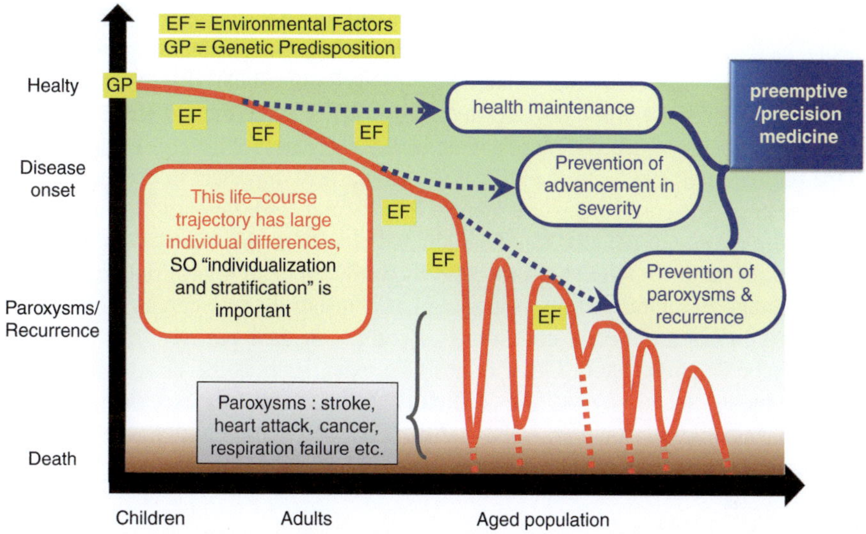

Fig. 5.2 A new concept of disease prevention, "preemptive/precision medicine". This is a new concept of disease prevention based on the principle of "medical science for individuals," which stratifies/individualizes high-risk diseases and forecasts the disease onset, advancement in severity, paroxysms, and recurrence with a high probability through the use of genetic predisposition, biomarker, clinical information, social data, etc., in addition to establishing appropriate preventive intervention (improvement of lifestyles (meals, physical exercise, etc.), pharmaceuticals, etc.) according to the risks

First, depending on the type of each disease, the process leading to the onset/advancement in severity/paroxysm and recurrence of the disease differs. Therefore, it needs to be identified what type of how intense risk factors exist at which period of a person's life in an exhaustive manner (e.g., genetic predisposition, biomarker, clinical data, social data, etc.). Then it is necessary to analyze those factors in chronological order, establish high-precision "forecasting" technology, and stratify/individualize the persons on an appropriate scale from the viewpoints of economy, safety, and effectiveness. And finally, by establishing highly cost-effective intervention technology (for lifestyles (meals, physical exercise, etc.), pharmaceuticals and so on) according to the "forecast" result of each disease, prevention of the onset/advancement in severity/paroxysm and recurrence of the disease.

In order to establish these technologies, strategic R&D integrating various fields concerning life science and medical science is required. In recent years, important scientific insights likely to be a key to realizing "preemptive/precision medicine" have been noted one after another. In this document, while paying attention to the viewpoint of "DOHaD" as one of those insights, I describe the unified strategy for realizing "preemptive/precision medicine."

5.1.5 *Overview of DOHaD*

In realizing "preemptive/precision medicine" [4, 5], DOHaD (Developmental Origins of Health and Disease) [6] gives an important indication. DOHaD is a significant insight found through the research on birth cohorts, etc., conducted over the past few decades in Europe. DOHaD has shown in many instances the correlation of environmental factors (nutritional status, etc.) during the period from the fetal stage to infancy with obesity in childhood and at later stages, cardio-metabolic diseases (diabetes, cardiovascular disease, etc.), developmental disorder, mental disease, etc. These diseases are projected to become more and more serious issues for the entire human race in the future, and R&D focused on DOHaD will be very important in the future.

In the past, preventive measures against obesity and cardio-metabolic diseases in Japan were mainly targeted at middle-aged and elderly people who looked healthy. On the other hand, DOHaD has indicated the importance of appropriate care from the fetal stage to infancy. Moreover, going back further than the fertilization stage, the environments and health conditions of parents in their puberty (e.g., obesity, etc.) may be important, too. Other issues also exist, such as the lack of measurement/diagnosis technologies, the difficulty of intervention experiments, etc. However, in future research on disease prevention, it will be significant to incorporate the viewpoint of DOHaD.

5.1.6 Significance of Implementing DOHaD Research in Japan

Representative risk factors found through the cohort analyses in Europe include undernutrition of pregnant women, low birth weight of babies, age of women when they give birth, etc. Compared with those in other developed countries, Japanese women have a high proportion of thinness (suggestive of undernutrition) [7]. Also influenced by the concept of "have a small baby and raise it to grow big" peculiar to perinatal care in Japan, the proportion of low birth weight babies is high [8]. Additionally, in association with women's activated participation in the society, the average age of marriage has increased coupled with childbearing age. These facts show the possibility that babies in Japan have a high risk of disease from birth. Thus, there is an urgent need for strategic R&D focused on DOHaD in this country.

The presence of ethnic differences also needs to be noted. DOHaD research is led by European countries, but European countries differ from Japan in the genetic predisposition of people, environmental factors, medical systems, etc. Therefore, insights obtained in the European region cannot be applied as they are to Japanese people. In fact, their life span, body shapes, disease patterns, etc. are considerably different. For this reason, we need to immediately build up scientific evidence targeting Japanese people.

5.2 R&D Strategy for "Preemptive/Precision Medicine (Including DOHaD)"

First, we should establish epidemiological research bases (cohort, data of the administration, etc.), and we should pursue the collection, management, and utilization of data. Considering the continuity with the data collected in the past and the latest

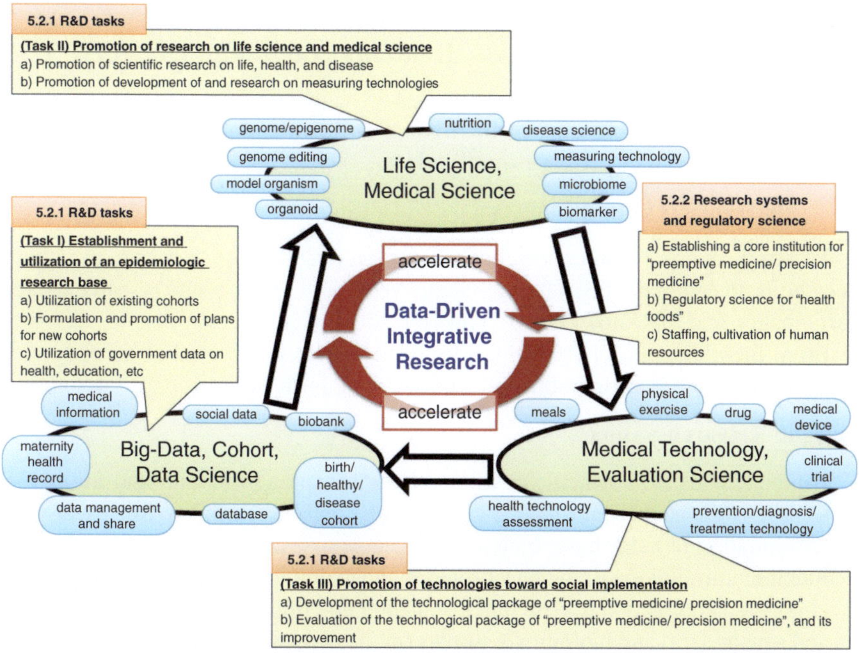

Fig. 5.3 An overall image of R&D subjects

knowledge, etc., we should specify important items for collection and collect data from a long-term point of view in a flexible manner. Hypothesis found in the epidemiology research base will lead to the clarification of detailed mechanisms through life science and medical science research, and new hypothesis found during the process should be verified on the basis of the epidemiology research base. By accelerating these cycles, a lot of scientific knowledge will be obtained, and development of the technological package of "preemptive/precision medicine" will progress significantly. In parallel with these, we will need to promote evaluation and research activities on the impacts on the economy, society, and people's health. Then, on the basis of the evaluation results, an optimal technological package should be established. We will identify new hypothesis from the data obtained through their use by many people in society and further promote life science and medical science research. It is an important issue to accelerate these data-driven researches, "IoBMT (Integration of Bio-Medical Things)."

The main direction of research on "preemptive/precision medicine" is as stated above. The main subject of this document, i.e., DOHaD, is one of the important approaches to research on "preemptive/precision medicine." I will describe specific R&D subjects, research systems, and regulatory science that should be pursued in Japan in the future (Fig. 5.3).

5.2.1 *R&D Tasks that Should Be Established in Japan ("Preemptive/Precision Medicine (Including DOHaD)")*

(Task I) Establishment and utilization of an epidemiologic research base: Collection and sharing of high-quality data

(a) **Utilization of existing cohorts.**

Existing cohorts (birth cohort, healthy person cohort, disease cohort, etc.) have been built up and maintained through many years of work by many researchers and participants, and this knowledge should be made the most of.

From the viewpoint of DOHaD, a lot of insights are expected of an integrated analysis on the information obtained from existing birth cohorts.

Specific Research Subjects

- Establishment of a system for integratively managing the data and biological samples collected from existing cohorts with high accessibility for researchers [compilation of a database, biobanking].
- Flexible introduction of the latest science and technology and insights in existing cohorts and collection of data (environmental and lifestyle data, personal device, and sensor data) and biological samples (medical records, genome, metabolome, microbiome, etc.) with higher values on the basis of the sufficient agreement of the participants.
- Collection of various social data (family environment, parent-child relationship, occupation, annual income, mental stress, etc.) on the basis of the sufficient agreement of the participants.

(b) **Formulation and promotion of plans for new cohorts.**

If some important data items or biological samples exist that are hard to obtain from existing cohorts, new cohorts shall be established on the basis of sufficient discussions and careful planning.

From the viewpoint of DOHaD, birth cohort and prenatal cohort (from pregnant women, etc.) are expected to be established. However, as such efforts will incur a huge cost, careful preparation is required (Refer to *[Column 1]*).

Specific Research Subjects

- Implementation of experimental efforts concerning small-scale cohorts (e.g., introduction of wearable devices) and practical efforts for larger cohorts to be extracted.
- Promotion of cohort research targeting events expected to result in a lot of small-scale benefits (pregnancy diabetes, natural pregnancy cases/pregnancy cases supported by assisted reproductive technology, etc.) and analytical research on the data thus obtained.
- Formulation and implementation of large-scale and long-term birth cohort plans (→It is required to have detailed discussions on various expert groups

(epidemiology, life science, medical science, economics, sociology, ethics, pedagogy, etc.) as well as detailed plans on data collection items, promotion system, procurement of long-term operating funds, etc.)

(c) **Utilization of government data on health, education, etc. (including maternity health record books, etc.)**

In Japan, a huge amount of data already exists on health/education, etc., collected by administrative organs. Although there are issues concerning the difference in competent administrative entities and insufficient standardization of data items, etc., the data is still a mountain of treasure and should be made the most of.

From the viewpoint of DOHaD, a lot of knowledge is expected to be obtained through integrated analysis on the data from "maternity health record books," with a history of more than half a century and clinical information.

Specific Research Subjects

- Conversion of various data collected by administrative organs for health/education, etc., into a structured data that allows for integrated AI analysis (curation, standardization, etc.), and compilation of a database on maternity health record books, babies and infants, medical checkup for school children, and medical checkup/measurement of physical fitness/achievement test, electronic chart, statement of medical expenses, medical information, etc., during compulsory education, etc.
- Unification of various data at the national and local authority levels (annual income, family structure, demographic statistics, etc.), compilation of a database, and establishment of a system for appropriately sharing the data.
- Integrated analysis on the data obtained from existing various cohorts and the data from "maternity health record books".
- Acceleration of the digitalization of maternity health record books (It will be an interface for the social implementation of not only data collection methods but also the results of research on DOHaD.)

[Column 1] Studies toward the maintenance and development of longer-term cohorts, biobank, and database

By maintaining cohorts, biobanks, and databases for a long time, over 30–50 years, as the research base and keeping on developing them, their scientific and industrial significance will increase.

As cohorts, biobanks, and databases require a huge amount of labor, time, and cost for establishment and maintenance, a detailed promotion plan is essential. First, we will need to closely survey related trends in and out of the country and hold discussions among all stakeholders of Japan's industrial, academic, and governmental organizations, etc., for 3–5 years. Then, in consideration of the forecast of related technological fields and social needs, etc., in a comprehensive manner, a promotion plan will need to be formulated from a long-term point of view. Experts having strong leadership to put the plan into practice are needed to supervise all the activities and start the implementation phase at an optimal time.

For example, it is expected that the latest scientific knowledge in respect of data collection items and collection methods (wearable devices, innovative analytical technologies, new candidates for disease markers, etc.) will be reflected in cohorts. At the same time, in order to maintain the follow-up rate of cohorts, we need to develop a trusting relationship with cooperating people in respect of cohorts (active communication, appropriate information transmission, etc.). In addition, we should also pay attention to the trend of the individual medical number system scheduled to be introduced in 2020, the electronic health record, etc., which is expected to come into existence sooner or later. Moreover, it is also essential to respond to major changes in these infrastructures for science and technology and medical treatment and to correct the plan flexibly while maintaining the compatibility with collected data.

These efforts require government investment at their incipient stage, but it is unrealistic in the environment of an increasingly tightened national budget to depend only on national funds for a long time. Operating the systems with various financial sources will not only increase their robustness as infrastructures but also make the cohorts, biobanks, and databases worthy of being relied on by various sectors in and out of the country. One of the conceivable directions will be for the would-be beneficiary companies (pharmaceutical, food, insurance companies), organizations (health insurance associations), the government (not a single ministry or agency but multiple ministries, agencies, or government organizations), etc., to bear the operating cost under the condition that they provide knowledge and information thus acquired. We should also immediately start discussions on these frameworks for securing medium- to long-term budgets.

Meanwhile, new trends are emerging, too. For example, a US insurance company (Kaiser Permanente) is proceeding with the compilation of a database and biobank of various information about insured people, while a US genome analysis company (23andMe) is proceeding with the establishment of a large-scale database focused on the genome information of its hundreds of thousands of customers. At present, the scale of the activities of private companies corresponding to these is still small in Japan, but it is expected to significantly expand in the future. While adequately grasping these trends in the private sector, we should discuss and implement the desirable division of roles and linkage in relation to the bases built up by the government.

The above efforts will be an asset to Japan in the future. And further, they will be the source of competition in R&D and will be the backbone of evidence for policy-making.

(Task II) Promotion of research on life science and medical science: Deepening the understanding of life

(a) **Promotion of scientific research on life, health, and disease.**

In order to use the results of research on "preemptive/precision medicine" for commercialization, it is desirable to pursue research on humans. However, it takes a long time for a seemingly healthy person to show signs of a disease or have a paroxysm. Therefore, in actual cases, research using biological samples of model animals or humans (in DOHaD, placenta, umbilical cord blood, the body fluid of pregnant women and babies/infants (blood, urine), etc.) will need to be promoted.

Then, by carrying out an integrated analysis on the knowledge obtained this way with the data acquired from the abovementioned epidemiology base, the knowledge is refined to a highly extrapolated one for humans.

From the viewpoint of DOHaD, the following are two particularly notable topics. One is that it is noted from research on model animals that an epigenome is inherited across generations. This is an important finding which indicates the need to go back further than the fetal stage (to a period before pregnancy, puberty, etc., of the parent) of the relevant person in order to provide adequate preventive measures against a disease. It is expected that more intellectual bases will be built up in the future. The other is that a relationship between microbiome (intestinal flora, etc.) and the child is indicated, in relation to which the Bill & Melinda Gates Foundation has initiated a global effort to start the long-term follow-up of cohorts, etc. Research on microbiomes has also been activated in Japan, and further activation of research on microbiomes targeting the period from fetal stage to infancy is expected [9].

Specific Research Subjects

(1) Development of experimental methods.

- Development and sustainment of model animals making the most of genome-editing technologies (CRISPR/Cas9), etc.
- Development of simulation technologies (simulation of organs/fetuses, the process from birth to aging, inheritance to the next generation (of epigenomes, etc.), the process of evolution of model animals and humans, etc.)
- Use of organism species having peculiar physiology as experimental animals (killifish (short lived), naked mole rat (showing no symptoms of aging), etc.)
- Development of human *in vitro* experiment systems (organoids originating from human cells, organ-on-a-chip, etc.)

(2) Promotion of research on epigenome/genome.

- Elucidation of the mechanism of intergenerational transmission of epigenome (from parents, grandparents, great grandparents, etc.)
- Elucidation of the mechanism of change in epigenomes caused by environmental factors influencing birth and aging and association with phenotypes.
- Elucidation of the relationship between the change in epigenomes during the fetal stage, infancy, and the subsequent process of growth and the disease onset mechanism; exploration of biomarkers/intervention methods.
- Promotion of research on genomes (identification of epigenome-related genes, genes having disease onset risks, etc.)

(3) Promotion of research on nutrition science.

- Identification of the nutrients involved in the change in epigenomes and elucidation of both the physiological significance and the metabolic mechanism.
- Elucidation of the relationship between the profile of microbiomes (intestinal flora), nutrition, metabolism, and exploration of improvement methods.

- Exploration of biomarkers/intervention methods, including the working mechanism of disease nutrients believed to be associated with the onset of diseases and related molecules.
- Elucidation of the influence of excess or deficiency in energy and nutrients, etc. (protein, amino acid, iron, folic acid, etc.), during the period from the fetal stage to infancy on the development/growth and the health condition after maturity, as well as elucidation of the working mechanism and exploration of biomarkers/intervention methods, including involved molecules.
- Establishment of a simple and accurate method of collecting and analyzing data on meals (collection of and analysis on data taken with a smartphone camera and so on).

(4) Promotion of scientific research on diseases.

- Exploration of candidates for biomarkers/treatment technologies on the basis of a disease onset mechanism.
- Acceleration of research on the period from the fetal stage to baby/infant stages by making the most of a host of scientific knowledge accumulated through past scientific research on diseases (onset mechanisms, biomarkers, etc.) (e.g., comparative study on diseases showing similar pathology in babies and infants).

(b) **Promotion of development of and research on measuring technologies.**

The driving force of technology development for "preemptive/precision medicine" is high-quality big data, and measurement technologies for data collection are placed at an important position. It is believed that there are two environments for data collection, i.e., daily data collection using wearable devices and data analysis during medical checkup/examination using precision measuring technologies, each of which requires R&D.

Additionally, from the viewpoint of DOHaD, measuring technologies for fetuses (babies and infants) is likely to be the largest bottleneck. First, since the technologies that can be used to measure the state of fetuses are limited, data on fetuses is especially deficient. In order to realize the improvement of the intrauterine environment on the basis of scientific evidence, a breakthrough is required for measuring and analyzing technologies. When compared with the cases of adults, measurement and analysis of babies and infants involve many challenges, and a more minimally invasive (noninvasive), rapid, and simple measuring method is essential. As both noninvasiveness and ease in measurement are strongly required for the measuring technologies for fetuses, babies, and infants, the established technologies are expected to be developed and applied not only to fetuses, babies, and infants but also to adults, the aged population, etc.

Specific Research Subjects

(1) Development of ultrahigh-precision measurement/analytical technologies and daily data collection/analytical technologies.

- Measurement/analytical technologies for infinitesimal body fluid (blood, urine, saliva, etc.)

- Development of wearable devices (development of sensing technologies, data processing/communication technologies, and data analysis technologies).

(2) Development of measurement/analysis technologies for the state of fetuses.

- Promotion of research on the improvement/sophistication of electrocardiogram for fetuses, implementation of programs for the dissemination of related technologies.
- Development of measurement/analysis technologies for the various parameters of fetuses (blood pressure and pulse wave of fetuses, measurement/evaluation of the growth state in the womb, etc.)
- Development of measurement/analysis technologies for substances contained in maternal blood originating from fetuses (DNA, mRNA, epigenome, protein, lipid, sugar chain, microRNA, etc.)

(3) Development of measurement/diagnosis technologies for the state of babies and infants.

- Development of measurement/diagnosis technologies and minimally invasive (noninvasive), rapid, and simple sampling (painless blood sampling, oral cells, secreted sebum, hair root, and others).
- Development of quantitative evaluation technologies for the state of development and growth.
- Development of innovative measurement/diagnosis technologies (e.g., developmental disorder (autism spectrum disorder, etc.))

(Task III) Promotion of technologies toward social implementation: Sophistication of technologies and dissemination/wider use of them across society

(a) **Development of the technological package of "preemptive/precision medicine" (evaluation/intervention technologies for disease risk).**

By analyzing the big data acquired through the efforts of the abovementioned "Task I", "Task II" and the latest scientific knowledge in an integrated manner and verifying/sophisticating the technologies thus developed, evaluation/intervention technologies for disease onset risk essential for the social implementation of "preemptive/precision medicine" technologies shall be established.

In general, the contribution of each disease risk factor to the onset of a disease is low. In order to enhance the precision of evaluation/intervention models for disease onset risks, it will be effective to carry out analyses focused on multiple disease risk factors and their time series variation. On the other hand, the only approach of Fisher statistics under the assumption of a huge parent population in conventional large-scale randomized trials, etc., by itself has limitations. It is expected that after recognizing a certain degree of uncertainty by making the most of the approach of Bayesian statistics, the number of analyzed cases will gradually be increased and a higher precision evaluation/intervention model for disease onset risks will be established.

Artificial intelligence technology can be noted as a remarkable trend in recent years. At present, efforts aiming to formulate diagnosis/treatment plans using

Watson (of IBM) having advanced machine learning and reasoning functions have been initiated and led by the USA. Additionally, deep learning technologies are attracting a great deal of attention throughout the world. These artificial intelligence technologies have a potential to dramatically accelerate both the development of the technological package of "preemptive/precision medicine" and its social implementation. These artificial intelligence technologies, however, should be appropriately introduced and utilized after identifying the potential of such technologies.

From the viewpoint of DOHaD, the improvement of the intrauterine environment through nutritional improvement, etc., for pregnant women, I believe, will be effective for them (fetuses) as a specific intervention method. In the period of babies/infants and subsequent stages, it will be possible to adopt less invasive methods (improvement of eating lifestyles (meals, physical exercise, etc.)) for smaller onset risks and rather invasive methods for larger disease onset risks (intake of specified nutrients or adequate administration of pharmaceuticals).

Specific Research Subjects

(1) Data groups, etc., required for analyses.

- Extraction of correlation and rules, estimation of the relation between causes and effects, analytical research on major factors, etc., should be conducted for the large-scale time series data groups concerning the health maintenance/disease risk factors acquired from the abovementioned "Task I.": the data groups are as follows:
  - Biological data. Genome information, biochemistry information (protein, metabolites, etc.), vital information (blood pressure, etc.), image information (MRI, etc.) markers, etc.
  - Life data. Meals, physical exercise, life rhythm, the situation of exposure to environmental chemicals, etc.
  - Governmental data groups on health and education, etc. Annual income, family structure, occupation, data on maternity health record books, data on medical checkups for school children/babies and infants, medical checkup/measurement of physical fitness/achievement test during compulsory education, etc., medical checkup data of companies, electronic charts, statement of medical expenses, etc.
- A wide variety of scientific knowledge on health maintenance/disease risk factors acquired by abovementioned "Task II."
  - Knowledge on various vital phenomena: epigenome, nutrition science, behavioral science, biogenesis science, aging science, metabolic science, homeostatic mechanism, microbiome (intestinal flora, etc.)

(2) Development of the technological package of "preemptive/precision medicine" (evaluation/intervention technologies for disease onset risks).

- Analyses incorporating the concept of time series on multiple disease risk factors, sophistication of prevention/diagnosis/treatment technology seeds.

  - Development of integrated analytical technologies for multilayered and multidimensional information.
  - Development of an optimal designing method for clinical research/tests (through the use of Bayesian statistics, etc.)
  - Development and implementation of new bioinformatics technology including artificial intelligence (deep learning technology, etc.)

- Optimal stratification of target groups according to health condition and disease type and establishment of preventive intervention technologies (including the unification of evaluation/diagnosis technologies and intervention technologies).

  - Stratification technologies: Health condition evaluation markers, onset forecasting markers, diagnostic equipment.
  - Preventive intervention technologies: Chemical compounds for improving health condition, pharmaceuticals, new drug modalities (fecal microbiota transplantation, microbial cocktail technology, etc.), digital theraphy (smart phone app), medical equipment, etc.

(b) **Evaluation of the technological package of "preemptive/precision medicine" (health, economic, and social impacts) and its improvement.**

In order to realize a better society through the implementation of technologies, health, economic, and social impacts of the technological package of "preemptive/precision medicine" (mentioned in "Task III-a") need to be evaluated.

In general, short-term and direct effects of disease prevention are hard to see. In particular, as DOHaD takes a long time until the disease onset, this tendency is remarkable in this case. Therefore, efforts to quantitatively visualize the health, economic, and social impacts as much as possible through the prevention of those diseases are extremely important in respect of the following two points.

1. It can be verified in advance how significant the relevant technology is in the medium- to long-term from the viewpoint of people's health/national finances/industries.
2. Development of motivation and change of actions can be expected when the technological impacts are conveyed to the stakeholders of the people, researchers, administrative officers, health-care providers, etc., in an understandable manner.

Specific Research Subjects

(1) Establishment of technologies for evaluating health, economic, and social impacts.

- Refinement of methods for evaluating medical technologies currently used for calculating the standard prices for new medicines.

  - More efficient analyses on a large amount of data and research on modeling as a method that can complement deficient data for analyses (e.g., decision tree model, Markov model, Monte Carlo simulation, etc.)

- Research for evaluating the health outcome of medical technologies (e.g., cost-benefit analysis (willingness to pay, social cost, etc.), cost-utility analysis (e.g., QALY (product of QOL and years of life), patient-reported outcome).
- Research evaluating clinical economy (e.g., cost minimization analysis, cost-effectiveness analysis, cost-benefit analysis, cost-utility analysis, cost-of-illness analysis, cost-consequence analysis, etc.)

• Development of a method for evaluating the "preemptive/precision medicine technology," which can be thought of as far more complicated than the calculation of standard prices for medicines: examples of components that need additional analyses.

  - Life expectancy and QOL that can be improved by disease prevention (including the change in QOL and time cost of not only the relevant person but also his/her family members, etc.)
  - Influences on medical expenses and care expenditure (implementation cost of the "preemptive/precision medicine" technology, medical expenses involved in diseases that can be controlled by disease prevention, and those expected to occur in the future).
  - Social cost (loss of opportunities for the work of the relevant persons, social activities, cultivation of the young, etc.)
  - Sense of values of the people (social agreement status, etc., of health/medical care, bioethics, etc.)

(2) Evaluation (health, economic, and social impacts) and improvement of the package of "preemptive/precision medicine".

  • Carry out evaluation from the development stage of the technological package of "preemptive/precision medicine" and accelerate the development, correct the direction of technologies, or stop the development. The evaluation method is immature under the circumstances, but by continuing the evaluation in actual fields, the evaluation method can be expected to be established early.

[Column 2] Expectations for pharmaceutical companies

Pharmaceuticals, food (nutrients), etc., are positioned as specific important intervention technologies for "preemptive/precision medicine." In developing these technologies, we set high expectations for pharmaceutical companies.

At present, pharmaceutical companies are mainly engaged in activities for developing diagnostic methods and treatment methods. However, drug development faces many difficulties such as the lack of promising drug discovery targets, a decline in development success rate, complication of manufacturing processes, more strict examination by regulatory bodies, etc. As a result, soaring prices of new pharmaceuticals cannot be contained, and this has become a factor that puts pressure on government finances. The conventional-type pharmaceutical development model which had grown for several decades has already collapsed. In such a situation, one of the possible responses for the time being would be to make the R&D process more efficient through the use of ICT (supercomputers, AI, Health Tech). However, pharmaceutical companies should pursue not only a more efficient process but also a larger market scale.

In the future, pharmaceutical companies should try to convert themselves to health-care companies engaged in "preemptive/precision medicine." This is a new challenge into the area of "prevention" that pharmaceutical companies haven't tried to address in the past, and the following two points will lead to success, I believe.

(a) *Building up an infrastructure for collecting evidence concerning "prevention" – real-world data.*

It is difficult to collect evidence for "prevention" through large-scale randomized trials. When a parent population is created for "prevention" on the basis of Fisher statistics, we will need to follow up a huge parent population of a million to ten million people for a long time, inevitably incurring considerable costs, which will be unrealistic. A promising alternative would be to use "big data." The quality of data is what matters most to extract appropriate results from big data.

In such case, pharmaceutical companies will be required to coordinate with ICT companies and the government and to collect various data on the health and diseases of people (including the use of wearable devices). Then, analytical technologies for big data (Bayesian statistics, artificial intelligence technology, etc.) will need to be sophisticated. A research infrastructure that will make possible the collection and use of such data will be the source of the competitive capacity for creating "prevention" technologies in the future.

(b) *Development of prevention technologies.*

New ideas for "prevention" technologies should be sought from free and creative research in academia. As a role of pharmaceutical companies, the importance of strategic R&D investments aimed at academia and the judgment for promising "preemptive/precision medicine" seeds will increase further. Additionally, developments for commercialization and evaluation tests/clinical research pharmaceutical companies are skillful at will maintain their importance. Research at the precompetitive stage such as the establishment of safety markers, etc., required for evaluation tests will be effectively carried out through the joint research platform system composed of multiple pharmaceutical companies, regulatory agencies, etc., in a unified fashion.

5.2.2 Research Systems and Regulatory Science that Should Be Established in Japan

(a) Establishing a core institution for "preemptive/precision medicine".

Compared with conventional-type R&D on treatment, the research on "preemptive/precision medicine" takes longer. The time lag from the time when a symptom emerges until the disease onset, advancement in severity or paroxysm, etc., is considerably different depending on the disease involved. For example, while the time from symptom onset to a paroxysm tends to be shorter in the case of cardiovascular disease, the time length for dementia and diabetes tends to be longer, i.e., several years to several 10 years.

Therefore, research should also be pursued from a medium- to long-term point of view. In addition, a core institution to promote such research with a sense of mission and responsibility should be established. Such a core institution is required to set priority issues from a medium- to long-term point of view and to carry out cross-cutting R&D beyond the confines of the relevant domestic ministries and offices. Maximization of the research results will be expected as a whole if each region of the country promotes research in competition for new ideas and the progress is grasped and coordinated by the core institution. Moreover, the core institution is also expected to make active efforts for establishing a system of cooperation between Japan and Europe, the USA, China, etc.

(b) Regulatory science for "health foods".

As for "health foods," discussions on regulatory science as one of the disease prevention technologies are required. In recent years, regulations on "health foods" have been enacted in Japan one after another. However, the "health foods" meeting the minimum rules of the current regulations can't be expected to enhance people's QOL in an ensured manner.

The "health foods" industry is, like the automobile industry, the household electrical industry, etc., one of the industries Japan has strength in. People can directly feel the usability in the case of devices and components like automobiles, refrigerators, smartphones, etc. On the other hand, the effect of "health foods" often depends on the advertising statements of companies, and people can't easily feel their direct usability when compared with the abovementioned devices and components. For this reason, strict regulations should be enacted, and related products should be approved only when the companies concerned respond to the genuine wish of people to be "in good health." Further, a system should be established to allow only those "health foods" actually having preventive effects be delivered to people.

(c) Staffing develop of human resources.

There is a considerable lack of experts in big data and research on epidemiology. Research on epidemiology requires human resources familiar with the know-how of establishing cohorts and maintaining a high follow-up rate for a long time. In addition, like research on epidemiology and life science, etc., all research is flooded with big data. We will need to cultivate and secure bioinformaticians who can analyze such big data appropriately and find meaningful results.

The type of human resources Japan decisively lacks is researchers evaluating health, the economy, and society impacts. It is essential to appropriately evaluate such health, economic, and social impacts for the sustainable development of our society in the future. As a place for cultivating human resources, it will be possible to set up a university, etc., providing courses in public health. Development of better methodologies and case studies should be promoted in universities under the leadership of Japanese or foreign experts specializing in the evaluation of medical technologies. In parallel with this effort, a system for reflecting evaluation results in national policies should be established, and the career paths (academic posts, administrative officials, R&D companies, think tanks, etc.) should be clarified.

At present, only a few Japanese researchers pursue research on DOHaD, being acutely aware of its significance. However, as the level of Japan's basic research on life science is world-class, this research is expected to attract many participants who recognize the importance of this field, and the world's top-level research will be advanced further.

5.3 Measures for the Social Dissemination of "Preemptive/Precision Medicine (Including DOHaD)"

5.3.1 Social Implementation of Research Results: A System for Fostering and Maintaining "Motivation"

At the start of the twenty-first century, R&D investments increased rapidly in Japan, and various disease prevention, diagnosis, and treatment technologies emerged. However, no better society will be realized just by establishing disease prevention, diagnosis, and treatment technologies. In Japan, effective disease prevention, diagnosis, and treatment technologies are not used appropriately for the enhancement of people's QOL, just like "pearls thrown before swine." R&D will be required also in the future. At the current stage, however, not just R&D, but a scheme for providing the results of R&D to people requiring them in an appropriate manner should be discussed and implemented in earnest.

An important keyword for the social dissemination of prevention is "motivation." Efforts to foster and maintain the "motivation" of both the provider side and the implementing side of prevention will be needed.

At present, it has become a serious issue in Japan that people having a chronic disease and attending hospital don't respect the drug administration rules laid down by the doctor (medication compliance). Reasons for this behavior may include "unintentionally forgetting to take the drug," "stopping to take the drug through the patient's own judgment," etc., but in the background lies technical problems in medication methods and the frequency, etc., as well as the lack of awareness of the disadvantages of not taking the drug, etc.

"Preemptive/precision medicine (including DOHaD)" targets the stage available for disease prevention. Therefore, compared with the abovementioned people having a chronic disease, it is more difficult to foster and maintain the "motivation" of these people not taking drugs. However, this problem cannot be avoided to realize a better society, and we will have to settle down to work on solving the problem.

In this section, I describe the "R&D" and the "establishment of a system" concerning "motivation," which, I believe, is the essence of disease prevention.

(a) R&D: pursuing stratification/individualization and convenience/usability.

Those involved in R&D should be acutely aware of the direction to foster and maintain people's "motivation."

In the past, general disease prevention methods for the people as a whole were to have adequate meals and physical exercise as well as to quit smoking, etc. While these are effective disease prevention methods, the problem was that only a part of the people who were highly conscious of disease prevention put them into practice. However, when a very safe and highly effective disease prevention technology stratifying/individualizing people is developed, "a highly effective disease prevention method you should carry out" will be clearly shown. Further, it will also show "yourself in the future" when you haven't carried out any prevention methods. As a result, many people will be able to recognize that prevention is an important issue you should address and carry out disease prevention with high motivation, I believe.

Various technology development paths can be conceived to maintain "motivation." For example, technology will be effective that allows the relevant person to feel a sense of accomplishment, such as by quantitatively visualizing the change in his/her physical constitution caused by disease prevention behavior with a biomarker, etc. Or, another disease prevention technology which provides a sufficient disease prevention effect by means of an easy-to-administer form (injection medicine, internal medicine, etc.) and a small number of administrations in a short term will also be effective. Moreover, in order to prevent a "failure in taking" disease prevention drugs, a different system will also be effective which automatically senses the completion or non-completion of drug administration and gives an alert, etc., when a "failure in taking" drugs occurs (e.g., ICT technology used for Abilify MyCite®). New technology called "digital medicine" has appeared, to realize healthcare management and prevention by smart phone application (e.g., Blue Star®)

(b) Systems: setting up a sustainable system, including incentivization for those concerned.

Social systems such as relevant schemes and regulations, etc., should be prepared for the provider side of prevention (industry, government, community, etc.) in order to allow the result of R&D to be delivered to each person.

Compared with general disease treatment methods, the short-term effects of prevention is invisible. Similarly, it will also be difficult, I believe, to feel the long-term effects, such as that "the relevant person wasn't taken ill." Incentivization will be required for each person to maintain high motivation and to carry out the methods steadily without getting tired of them. One direction for that purpose will be giving material or pecuniary rewards, commendations, etc., in each community provided on the basis of the evaluation of the effort and disease prevention behaviors of each person. However, ingenuity is required to prevent these rewards from being the very objective and to get people to understand that their health itself is the biggest reward of all in a skillful manner. For this purpose, it is important that the benefiting people understand disease prevention through education on health at various stages of their life, i.e., in high school, in university/college, in society, etc.

In the past, medical treatment was provided by medical institutions. However, for the purpose of prevention, elaborate and original efforts of various persons and organizations concerned will be expected, such as corporate health insurance societies, private insurers, pharmaceutical companies, health-care companies, etc. Activities not just depending on the government for financial resources and establishment of systems but involving the private sector will be a driving force for spreading disease prevention in the medium to long term.

[Column 3] Future form of the insurance system

The existence of the medical insurance system for the whole nation that Japan boasts is, conversely, also one of the factors for reducing the motivation for prevention. In the USA, 60% of all bankruptcies are caused by the inability to pay for medical expenses. In Japan, however, everyone can receive low-priced medical treatment. This fact has led to the tendency of people in Japan to feel that "Even if I should fall ill without paying attention to disease prevention and then the disease should worsen, I can visit the hospital and consult the doctor." The system of medical insurance for the whole nation should be maintained firmly in the future, but in respect of prevention, we should study a new framework for a different insurance system.

Here, I'd like to describe the medical insurance system for the whole nation, which is one of the social systems that can be involved in disease prevention. In the first place, the medical insurance system for the whole nation is a system established under the concept of supporting the medical expenses of people suffering from diseases by the whole nation contributing their share of the costs. (As a matter of fact, the financial resources depending only on the collection of insurance premiums are considerably insufficient, and a huge subsidy is provided from tax revenues.) However, since prevention targets almost all the people, it won't be appropriate that the system of medical insurance for the whole nation based on the spirit of mutual aid plays a central role in it. Moreover, it will also be unrealistic to make the government shoulder the burden of all costs of prevention, considering the tight financial condition. For this reason, the cost could be covered, for example, by private insurance. In that case, improvement of the profit of insurers is directly connected with the disease prevention behavior of the insured. For instance, it is conceivable as a method for the insured to provide information on disease prevention, to give rewards when disease prevention is successful, and to set up a scheme for adequately evaluating daily disease prevention behavior, reflecting the result in the insurance fee (implementing disease prevention = reduction of insurance fee), etc.

[Column 4] Stealth health care: What the next-generation public health ought to be

It is difficult to persuade everyone to change their behavior by just incentivizing prevention. On the other hand, sufficient evidence has been obtained, and "stealth health care" is effective as a disease prevention scheme that should be provided to everyone.

"Stealth health care" assumes a mechanism for everyone to carry out prevention activities unconsciously by incorporating prevention methods in social systems in a natural manner. To give an example, in the USA, while excessive consumption of

salt content has become an issue, it has been revealed that more salt content is contained in processed foods than in bottled table salt. To avoid the excessive intake of salt, it will be more effective to strengthen regulations on the use of salt in processed foods than to ask each of us to make an effort not to take too much salt in our everyday life. In the USA, from the viewpoint of DOHaD, nutrients that tend to be insufficient are selectively blended additionally under a food aid program for families on relief with pregnant women or infants.

As such a scheme involves incorporation in social systems and many people enjoy the fruits of such scheme unconsciously, collection of sufficient evidence and consensus building among those concerned are needed before introducing it. R&D and discussions for this purpose, I believe, will be important objectives Japan should pursue in the future.

5.4 Future Vision 2040

5.4.1 Life-Course Health Care

Here, I'd like to describe the future vision of health and medical care through 2040. The emerging central concept of "life-course health care" means physical and mental care from the viewpoint of the lifetime of humans. It is the direction Japan should pursue in the future to realize all social needs (enhancement of QOL, industrial vitalization, and optimization of medical expenses/care expenditure).

First, the entire genome information will be analyzed at the time of birth. Then, information on lifestyles (meals, physical exercise, etc.), biomarkers (molecules contained in the blood/urine and images), medical checkups, clinical information (electronic charts, statement of medical expenses, etc.), and so on is collected over a lifetime on a periodical basis. These data groups are managed in the domestic database. Under a management system which strikes a balance between security and convenience, academia, government, and companies proactively utilize the database. Analysis of the database not only deepens the understanding of life phenomena but also accelerates the R&D on "preemptive/precision medicine (including DOHaD)." The result of research will be provided to people not only through medical institutions but also through various organizations such as health insurance associations, private insurance companies, pharmaceutical and health-care companies, etc. It is expected that tips for further R&D can be obtained, and additional basic research will be developed when people actually comply with the principle of "preemptive/precision medicine (including DOHaD)."

By accelerating these cycles, a paradigm shift will occur from the current medical measures focused on cure (treatment, symptomatic therapy) to care (prevention of disease onset, prevention of advancement in severity, prevention of paroxysms and recurrence). Then, the targets for care will be increased from the past main target of the aged population to include the youth and from the viewpoint of DOHaD, babies, and infants. Additionally, even if "preemptive/precision medicine (including DOHaD)" progresses further, many people will face important issues like nursing care, the terminal phase, etc., sooner or later (*[Column 5]*). By also holding discussions on such matters and proceeding with consensus-building efforts, we will be able to realize physical/mental care from the standpoint of a lifetime, from before birth to the terminal phase, I believe.

[Column 5] How the terminal phase ought to be managed

Even if "preemptive/precision medicine (including DOHaD)" makes dramatic progress in the future and health problems are considerably improved, the "terminal phase" coming at the end of a lifetime cannot be avoided. We have many ups and downs in our lives in respect of health, social activities, human relations, etc., but "all's well that ends well."

In Japan, the response to the "terminal phase" has just begun. Since the latter half of the 2000s, formulation of guidelines has progressed rapidly on what terminal care ought to be, led by the societies for emergency medical services and palliative medicine, etc. In the future, we will need to carry out further activities recognizing consensus building in Japan and to make efforts, including legislation. In parallel with such rule-making efforts, it will also be important that each one of us prepare for the terminal phase of our lives at an early stage.

Approaches of science and technology are also effective for managing the "terminal phase." For example, by analyzing the big data on terminal care (electronic charts, etc.), it will be possible to measure the effect of terminal care, e.g., quantification of pain, etc. Additionally, various indications useful for terminal care will also be obtained from the huge amount of electronic charts of dead people (Figs. 5.4 and 5.5).

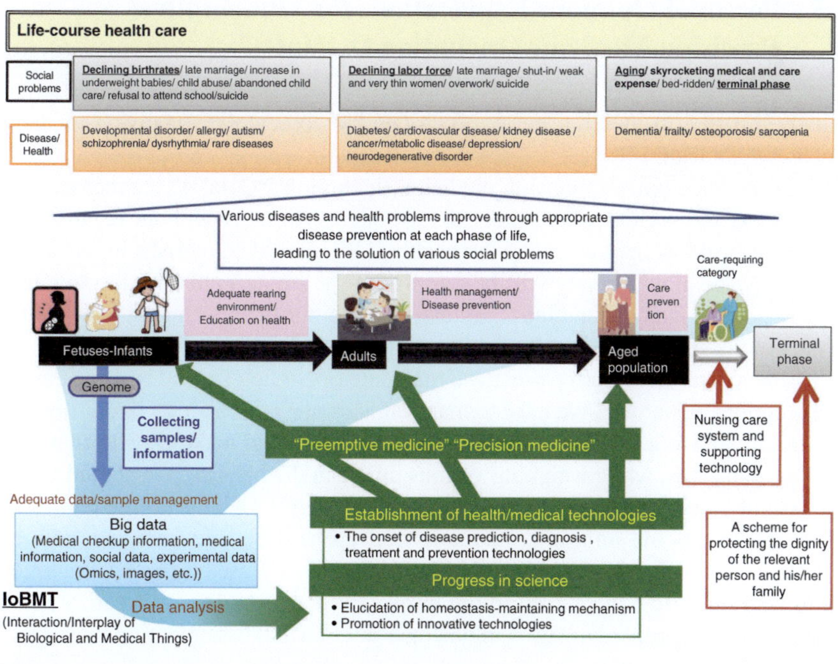

Fig. 5.4 Life-course health care (A future vision for 2040)

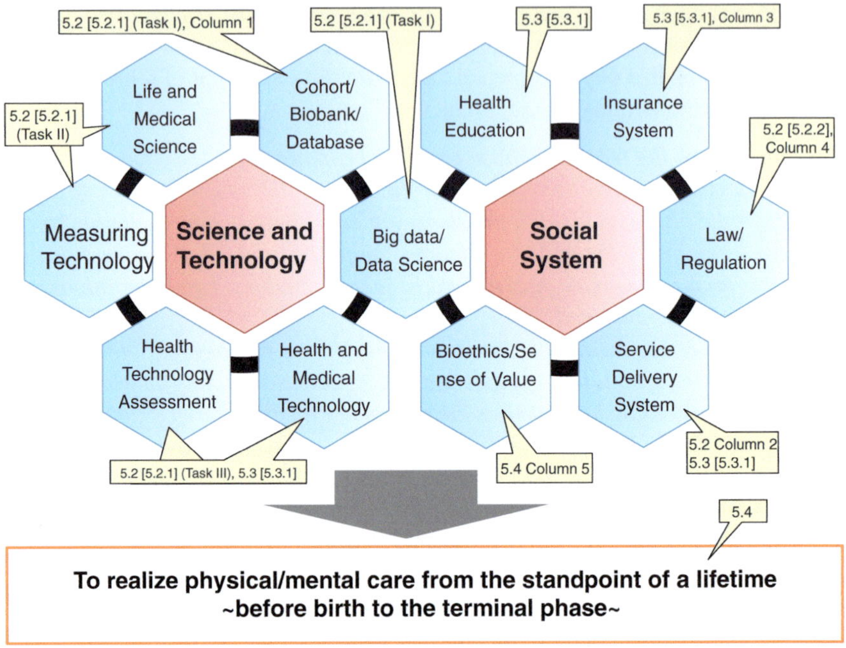

Fig. 5.5 Strategic framework to realize life-course health care

5.5 Personal Opinion: Expectations for "Preemptive/Precision Medicine (Including DOHaD)"

Finally, I'd like to mention my expectations for "preemptive/precision medicine (including DOHaD)."

Even if "preemptive/precision medicine (including DOHaD)" technologies are established, the society where these are introduced forcibly without regard to the intentions of the people would be "unhealthy." We should enjoy risks in our lives, I believe. A "healthy" society will be one where we are permitted to devote our all time to hobbies and occupations, eat tasty food to our heart's content, and indulge in dangerous amusements while risking somewhat unhealthy behavior.

I believe that "preemptive/precision medicine (including DOHaD)" is just one of many options in our life. We have to make choices one after another in our lifetime, and it will lead to a happy life, I believe, if we continue to make choices that seem best for ourselves, while weighing various things in the balance. We should not set the goal of "preemptive/precision medicine (including DOHaD)" to the realization of insipid health and long life. I hope its concept will be warm-hearted, with the primary objective being to support people's happy lives. Based on such recognition, I will lead Japan to a wonderful future through its R&D strategy for realization, as well as surveys, proposals, and implementation of social dissemination methods.

5.6 Conclusions

In order to realize "preemptive/precision medicine (including DOHaD)" and "life-course health care," we must implement various R&D themes and infrastructure development. But there is no time. Compared with the USA and the EU, it is hard to say that measures in Japan are progressing. We must implement them as soon as possible and open up a bright future for Japan. Therefore, as a member of Japan's public think tank organization, I would like to continue appealing to the government about the direction that science and technology policy should be.

Acknowledgments I wish to express my deep appreciation for the cooperation of Ms. Tsuneyo Nishino (Fellow, JST-CRDS), who gave a lot of valuable advice to me in writing this document. I'm very grateful to all my family members (Hirosato (3), Shin-Ichiro (5), and Akiko (37)) for their support. Meanwhile, please note that this document is published under the personal responsibility of the author, and it doesn't present the viewpoint of the affiliated organization.

References

1. Ministry of Health. Labour and Welfare homepage. http://www.mhlw.go.jp/
2. WHO. THE GLOBAL BURDEN OF DISEASE -2004 update, etc.
3. JST-CRDS. Strategic initiative: promotion of preemptive medicine in the Super-Aged Society. 2010.
4. JST-CRDS. Strategic proposal, promoting life course health-care: importance of preemptive medicine in pregnancy to child hood. Center for Research and Development Strategy; 2014.
5. The WHITE HOUSE PRESIDENT BARACK OBAMA "The Precision Medicine Initiative". 2015.
6. Gluckman PD, Hanson MA. Living with the past: evolution, development, and patterns of disease. Science. 2004;305:1733–6.
7. WHO. Global Database on Body Mass Index.
8. OECD. Health at a Glance 2011.
9. JST-CRDS. Strategic proposal, integrated promotion of human microbiome study: new development in life science and health care. 2016.

Part II
Public Health Aspect in Each Cohort or Consortium

Chapter 6
The ORIGINS Project

Erika Hagemann, Lyn Colvin, Lisa Y. Gibson, Sarah J. Miller, Debra J. Palmer, Ravisha Srinivas Jois, Desiree T. Silva, and Susan L. Prescott

E. Hagemann (✉) · L. Colvin
Telethon Kids Institute, University of Western Australia, Perth, WA, Australia

Edith Cowan University, Perth, WA, Australia
e-mail: erika.hagemann@telethonkids.org.au

L. Y. Gibson
Telethon Kids Institute, University of Western Australia, Perth, WA, Australia

Edith Cowan University, Perth, WA, Australia

University of Western Australia, Perth, WA, Australia

S. J. Miller · D. J. Palmer
Telethon Kids Institute, University of Western Australia, Perth, WA, Australia

R. Srinivas Jois
Edith Cowan University, Perth, WA, Australia

Joondalup Health Campus, University of Western Australia, Perth, WA, Australia

D. T. Silva
Telethon Kids Institute, University of Western Australia, Perth, WA, Australia

Edith Cowan University, Perth, WA, Australia

University of Western Australia, Perth, WA, Australia

Joondalup Health Campus, University of Western Australia, Perth, WA, Australia

S. L. Prescott
Telethon Kids Institute, University of Western Australia, Perth, WA, Australia

Edith Cowan University, Perth, WA, Australia

University of Western Australia, Perth, WA, Australia

Joondalup Health Campus, University of Western Australia, Perth, WA, Australia

DOHaD Society of Australia and New Zealand (Developmental Origins of Health and Disease), Australia, Southampton, UK

InVIVO Planetary Health, Worldwide Universities Network (WUN), Australia, West New York, NJ, USA

F. Sata et al. (eds.), *Pre-emptive Medicine: Public Health Aspects of Developmental Origins of Health and Disease*, Current Topics in Environmental Health and Preventive Medicine, https://doi.org/10.1007/978-981-13-2194-8_6

Abstract ORIGINS is a new birth cohort study, collecting detailed information about the early environment's influence on a broad range of non-communicable diseases. Over 5 years we aim to recruit 10,000 women and their partners early in pregnancy at Joondalup Health Campus (JHC) and collect biological samples, routine data and web-based questionnaires on their physical and mental health, diet, physical activity patterns and a range of factors in their environment, creating a large biobank and databank. We will intensively follow up these families until the children are 5 years of age. We will assess how early-life exposures influence child growth, development and health.

Nested within the main observational cohort will be a series of intervention studies to improve modifiable aspects of the early-life environment (e.g. nutrition, physical activity, microbial diversity and language development). ORIGINS is embedded in clinical care at JHC, and positive findings will be promptly translated into routine care for all families. Community and consumer representation is incorporated into this project. In addition to a dedicated ORIGINS Community Reference Group and Participant Reference Group, ORIGINS team members collaborate and participate with relevant local agencies, networks and groups. This encourages community engagement and provides avenues to disseminate information and findings to families and agencies.

ORIGINS will be a significant asset for the community as it has the potential to improve child and adolescent health and increase maternal, paternal, child and adolescent health research capacity, research productivity, research collaboration and translational impact.

Keywords Non-communicable diseases · Developmental Origins of Health and Disease (DOHaD) · Birth cohort · Interventions · Disease prevention · Community · Allergic disease · Immune development · Inflammation · Diet · Nutrition · Microbiome · Environmental pollutants · Gene-environment interactions · Obesity · Nature relatedness

Abbreviations

ADP	Air displacement plethysmography
AEDC	Australian Early Development Census
BENEFIT	Breastfeeding and Eating Nuts and Eggs For Infant Tolerance
CARE-Dads	Cardiovascular Risk Evaluation in Expectant Fathers
CDC	Child Development Centre
CRG	Community Reference Group
DOHaD	Developmental Origins of Health and Disease
ECU	Edith Cowan University
GA	Gestational age
GP	General practitioner
HREC	Human Research Ethics Committee

JHC	Joondalup Health Campus
MRC	Medical Research Council
NAPLAN	National Assessment Program—Literacy and Numeracy
NCDs	Non-communicable diseases
NHMRC	National Health and Medical Research Council
NIH	National Institutes of Health
PEA POD	Infant Body Composition System
PLAN	Pregnancy Lifestyle Activity and Nutrition
PRG	Participant Reference Group
RCT	Randomised controlled trial
RIGs	Research Interest Groups
SYMBA	Promoting gut health (symbiosis) with prebiotic fibre for prevention of allergic disease
TALK	Testosterone and Language in Kids
TEWL	Trans-epidermal water loss
TKI	Telethon Kids Institute
UWA	University of Western Australia
WA DoH	Western Australian Department of Health
WA	Western Australia
WAPHA	WA Primary Health Alliance
WHO	World Health Organisation

6.1 Introduction

The ORIGINS Project (ORIGINS, the Project) is a collaborative initiative between Joondalup Health Campus (JHC) and Telethon Kids Institute (TKI) to establish a new birth cohort in Western Australia (WA) that is fully integrated with clinical and diagnostic services and the community.

The development of many non-communicable diseases (NCDs), such as obesity, heart disease, allergies and poor mental health, can commence in utero or even preconception. The ORIGINS Project aims to uncover and understand when and why NCDs develop through the study of early-life environments, maternal and paternal physical and mental health and lifestyle, the microbiome, and genetics. The goal of ORIGINS is to reduce the rising epidemic of NCDs through 'a healthy start to life'.

A central objective of ORIGINS is to develop a comprehensive research platform through extensive databank and biobank facilities. This legacy project will provide a new platform to engage clinicians, researchers (across Australia and internationally), government and the wider community. Not only will ORIGINS enable world-class investigations into how, when and why NCDs develop, it will test early *interventions* to reduce the burden of these diseases. ORIGINS will be a pipeline for short-term productivity through a series of intervention studies, mechanistic studies, and targeted research. As well as facilitating strategic long-term research capacity, ORIGINS will be a 'responsive' system with 'real-time' feedback to parents and their children and translation to clinical and diagnostic services.

6.2 Hypothesis and Aims

The environment in pregnancy and early childhood determines physiological, structural, immune, metabolic and behavioural development and influences susceptibility to both early- and later-onset diseases [1]. Strategies to improve early-life environments are critical in reducing the rising global burden of chronic disease [2].

The specific aims of the ORIGINS Project are:

- To improve the health of the next generation through a better understanding of how to optimise the early environment.
- To generate a new birth cohort with a substantial databank and biobank to enable world-class research.
- To fully integrate the ORIGINS Project within the clinical framework of JHC.
- To initiate and integrate harmonised nested clinical trials within this framework.
- To understand the interaction of newly recognised exposures, such as the gut microbiome (not well studied in previous cohorts) of the mother and child as a key determinant of health and the risk of common NCDs (because of recognised immune, metabolic and neurodevelopment effects).
- To utilise new technologies (such as epigenetics, metagenomics, metabolomics, proteomics) and to understand the underlying mechanisms and pathways that lead to the current NCD burden.
- To harmonise with other major birth cohort studies, nationally and internationally, and to enable more collaborative work in the future, potentially allowing for the identification of risk factors in more rare health outcomes requiring large sample sizes [3].

6.3 Significance

The United Nations has identified the pandemic of NCDs as a major global threat and mandated development of preventive strategies that target common environmental risk factors. The inextricable link between the early environment and subsequent NCDs led the World Health Organisation (WHO) to prioritise 'early-life preventive strategies' [4–6]. Globally, health councils (such as NIH, MRC and NHMRC) now have 'a healthy start to life' as national priorities. To our knowledge, this is the first cohort study to examine how interventions with potential benefits on immune health, metabolic health and/or the microbiome may reduce inflammation in pregnancy and promote healthier outcomes of multiple organ systems.

ORIGINS directly addresses:

1. The call for integrated interdisciplinary studies to examine these complex interactions.
2. The Developmental Origins of Health and Disease (DOHaD) mandate to specifically target preventive strategies in early life.

6.4 A New Birth Cohort

The impetus for establishing a new birth cohort in WA is manifold. Changes in disease profile over the past two decades, with the emergence of new epidemics of early onset, surging rates of obesity, allergies, poor mental health and neurodevelopmental issues in young people, make a strong case for new cohorts to address these new challenges and establish a new profile of environmental risks [7].

The importance of newly recognised factors, such as the human microbiome, has not been investigated by previous birth cohort studies (without appropriate sample collections). Furthermore, advances in technology and improved data collections provide new opportunities to study new frontiers such as 'epigenetics' as critical mediators of genetic and environmental interactions during early development. This has prompted the need for new cohorts to collect new, early biological samples that are not available from older cohorts.

ORIGINS is following in the footsteps of two other internationally successful longitudinal cohort studies in Western Australia: the Raine Study and the Busselton Health Study. The Raine Study (http://www.rainestudy.org.au/) conducted recruitment from a Perth tertiary hospital between 1989 and 1991 ($N = 2868$ live births) and has been following up the cohort since, with the most recent follow-up of the cohort participants at age 27 (between 2016 and 2018). The Raine Study is one of the largest successful prospective cohorts of pregnancy, childhood, adolescence and now adulthood, to be carried out anywhere in the world. The Busselton Health Study (http://bpmri.org.au/) commenced in 1966 and conducted three yearly surveys of primary school children in Busselton in the southwest of Western Australia. Data has been collected from over 20,000 participants. Unlike ORIGINS, however, the Busselton Health Study did not collect early exposure information from pregnancy nor early childhood, while the Raine Study collected limited data on the environmental exposures in pregnancy. The ORIGINS Project is very much focused on this area and has the ability to look at epigenetic effects. The science has evolved greatly from 1966 to 1990 to present—the human genome has been mapped, and there is increasing interest on how the human microbiome impacts on health and immune responses in children. The Raine Study and Busselton Health Study were not able to collect or account for these important changes.

ORIGINS is unique and different from the Raine Study, the Busselton Health Study and other cohort studies where, in addition to observational data, this project will provide a framework for a series of smaller intervention studies that will be nested within the main observational cohort. Interventions will be focused on improving modifiable aspects of the early-life environment (such as nutrition, physical activity, time spent indoors and outdoors, smoking and pollutants, microbial diversity, water, air and food quality).

Over 5 years, the ORIGINS Project aims to recruit 10,000 pregnant women and their partners planning to deliver their baby at JHC. It is a project goal to recruit 5000 pregnant women (and their partners and children) as routine/non-active participants. Consent as a routine/non-active participant allows access to data collected during routine clinical care at JHC such as weight, height, blood pressure measurements, allergies, medications prescribed, glucose tolerance test result and routinely collected biological samples. It also allows ORIGINS access to records held at other health and allied services, e.g. immunisation records, GP records, hospital admissions in WA and data linkage to collections held by the Australian Government such as prescription medicines dispensed by pharmacies and childhood immunisation records. It is a project goal to recruit a further 5000 pregnant women (and their partners and children) as full/active participants. In addition to access to routine data, full/active participants agree to provide additional lifestyle and environmental data through a series of web-based questionnaires, biological sample collections and child clinic assessments. Initially these families will be intensively followed up until the children are 5 years of age.

6.4.1 The Databank

There are currently approximately 3700 deliveries per year at JHC, and over a 5-year period, we will integrate routine care data, collected on all patients delivering their baby at JHC, into the ORIGINS databank. For participants (mothers, partners and children) recruited into ORIGINS, we will seek consent for collection and storage of:

1. Routine data collected during routine clinical care at JHC.
2. Data linkage to WA and national data sets.
3. Web-based questionnaires and child clinic assessments.

The routine data collected during routine clinical care at JHC includes the JHC mother's and father's health questionnaire, the antenatal record, results and reports, such as results from the routine glucose tolerance test and routine anatomy ultrasounds, and all the information captured in the antenatal (Genie), birth and postnatal (Meditech and special care nursery database) JHC healthcare information management systems.

Data linkage to WA and national data sets will provide immunisation records, pathology results and prescription medicines collected through pharmacies; the Australian Early Development Census (AEDC) results, a national survey of children in their first year of school; the National Assessment Program—Literacy and Numeracy (NAPLAN) results, a national assessment of literacy and numeracy, measured at school; and notification of developmental anomalies through the WA Register of Developmental Anomalies.

Data relating to sleep, physical activity, diet and nutrition, lifestyle, mental health and wellbeing, skin and sun exposure, child health and development, demographics and social characteristics, medical history, neighbourhood and environment is collected through the web-based questionnaires. At the child clinic assessments, allergic disease symptoms and allergen sensitisation, skin barrier permeability, body size, body composition, developmental milestones, language,

Table 6.1 Summary of data collections for full/active participants

	Antenatal		Postnatal					Childhood						
	20 or 28 weeks	36 weeks	Birth	2 mths	4 mths	6 mths	9 mths	1 yr	1.5 yrs	2 yrs	2.5 yrs	3 yrs	4 yrs	5 yrs
CLINICAL ASSESSMENT														
PEA POD			C											
Bod Pod											C			C
TEWL		M						C			C			C
Skin prick test								C			C			C
Eczema assessment								C			C			C
Anthropometry								C			C			C
Developmental review								C			C			C
Developmental assessment**								C			C			
BIOBANK COLLECTIONS														
Blood	M, F	M						C			C			C
Urine	M	M			M, C	M, C		C			C			C
Buccal swab	M, F	M	F			M*, C*		M, C			C			C
Saliva	M, F	M	F		M*, C*	C*		M, C			C			C
Stool	M	M		M, C	M, C	M, C		C			C			C
House dust		M						M			M			M
Meconium			C											
Cord blood			C											
Cord tissue			C											
Placenta			C											
Colostrum			M											
Breast milk				M	M	M		M						
Hair	F	M						M, F						

*Only if seen in clinic at these time points for sub project appointments.
**Between 10 and 15% of the full/active participants, who are identified from the developmental review as requiring a more in-depth assessment, will return for a full developmental assessment and referral, by a paediatrician at the 1-year clinic check and a clinical psychologist at the 2.5-year clinic check

motor, behavioural, emotional and social development data are collected. These are measured and assessed through allergen skin prick testing, the PEA POD (measures body composition), the TEWL (trans-epidermal water loss) machine (useful in evaluating skin barrier permeability) and with a developmental review by a paediatrician. Between 10 and 15% of the participants who are identified as requiring a more in-depth assessment will return for a full developmental assessment and referral. A summary of the data collected in the child clinic assessments is detailed in Table 6.1.

6.4.2 *The Biobank*

Biobanks form essential components of a research program as they allow the investigation of novel factors, biomarkers and drug targets and associated factors in groups of patients that have been carefully categorised according to clinical status and outcome. Samples stored in biobanks can be utilised years after establishment, when new discoveries or technologies open up areas of research that were unimaginable when the samples were originally taken.

Modern biobanks are now recognised as important infrastructural platforms for specimen and data sharing not just as tools for single studies. Funding for research data, biological samples and the infrastructure needed to maximise their scientific utility is viewed as an investment that will benefit the public. This is illustrated by the recent joint statement of purpose issued by 17 major funders of health research, which endorses sharing data to improve public health [8].

The objectives of the ORIGINS biobank are:

- To provide a resource for research that is valued by society and conducted within applicable laws, regulations and ethical frameworks.
- To ensure the collection, storage, transfer, access and disposal of participants' biological samples are scientifically, legally and ethically appropriate.
- To secure the sustainability of the biobank, the protection of participants' privacy, the confidentiality of samples and ongoing public trust and involvement.

The ORIGINS biobank contains all the biological samples and the biological and genetic data that are generated from the samples collected from ORIGINS participants. Biological samples are collected from full/active participants at nine time points, from the first antenatal clinic visit (at approximately 20 or 28 weeks' gestation) until the child is 5 years of age. The collections include blood, saliva, buccal swab, stool, urine, house dust, hair, cord blood, cord tissue, placenta, meconium, colostrum and breast milk. A summary of the biobank collections is detailed in Table 6.1.

6.4.3 Project Governance

A governance framework has been developed for the project to accomplish governance, compliance and ethics. This framework outlines guiding principles for ORIGINS and provides a well-defined governance structure with roles and responsibilities clearly outlined, in addition to setting expectations and parameters for decision-making, management, reporting, scope and approval of nested sub projects. Refer to Fig. 6.1 for a diagrammatic schema of the ORIGINS governance structure.

The governance framework has been drafted in line with the collaboration agreement of the ORIGINS Project between TKI and JHC and based upon the NHMRC, *National Statement on Ethical Conduct in Human Research* [9].

Consumer and community representation is incorporated into the ORIGINS governance framework and structure to ensure that the community is fully engaged and informed with ORIGINS.

6.4.4 Nested Sub projects

ORIGINS is unique and different from other cohort studies where it provides a framework and governance structure for the nesting of intervention studies, randomised controlled trials and observational and mechanistic studies within the main

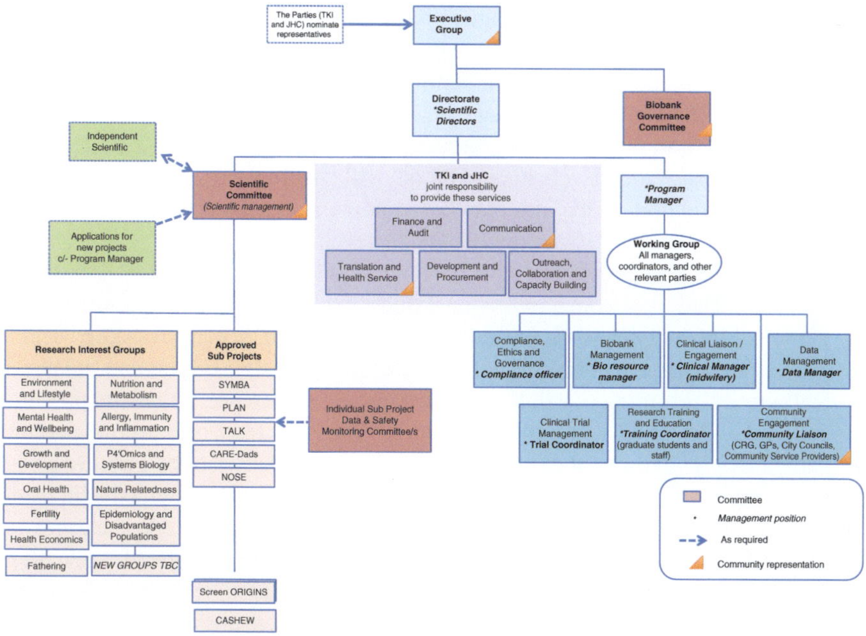

Fig. 6.1 ORIGINS governance structure

observational cohort. With their consent, all ORIGINS participants are screened to determine eligibility for sub projects. These nested sub projects, each with their own funding and Human Research Ethics Committee (HREC) approval, are strategically coordinated with ORIGINS, optimising on harmonised recruitment processes and harmonised 'outcomes' and 'exposures' data measures. This integrated approach allows more strategic interdisciplinary collaboration and coordinated follow-up with greater economies of scale with a more holistic multisystem approach to achieve a healthier start to life for the long-term health of the community.

Nine sub projects have already been approved by the ORIGINS executive. These are:

1. SYMBA: This is a double-blinded randomised controlled trial to examine the effects of maternal prebiotic supplementation in pregnancy and lactation on offspring outcomes of both clinical allergic disease and mechanistic immune development. Results of this study will directly inform allergy prevention recommendations. This study will generate new knowledge on the interactions between maternal diet, maternal microbiome and infant immune development.
2. PLAN: Pregnancy Lifestyle Activity and Nutrition

   The PLAN project is also a randomised controlled trial. It examined the feasibility of conducting a lifestyle (diet and physical activity) intervention starting in the first trimester of pregnancy, with the aim of promoting healthy gestational weight gain in early pregnancy. Controlling weight gain in pregnancy is likely to have a range of benefits to the babies born from these pregnancies. Even small changes in infant adiposity have the potential to change future obesity trajectory, leading to a lifetime of cost savings.

3. TALK: Testosterone and Language in Kids

   TALK is an observational study which follows women from 18 weeks' gestation until birth and then their child until 3 years of age to understand biological factors that may underpin language development. The data collected, including rate of growth in brain volume (through ultrasound at 18 and 24 weeks' gestation) and testosterone levels in cord blood, will enable the exploration of several hypotheses relating to the interplay between prenatal testosterone exposure and brain growth and their relation to language development.
4. CARE-Dads: Cardiovascular Risk Evaluation in Expectant Fathers

   CARE-Dads is also an observational study, but it is recruiting expectant fathers participating in ORIGINS to undergo a supplementary cardiovascular health evaluation comprising of a questionnaire regarding lifestyle behaviours and physical activity, recording of height, weight, waist circumference, and blood pressure and collection of an additional sample of blood for assay of cardio-metabolic parameters. The results will provide a cross-sectional snapshot of cardiovascular risk in men of reproductive age. Each participant will also be provided with feedback on their individual results and encouraged to adopt lifestyle measures to improve their health, with a follow-up questionnaire to be completed 1 year after the initial evaluation. This will facilitate future interventions to improve health of dads and ultimately increase the wellbeing of families as a whole.
5. NOSE pilot: a vulnerable airway epithelium—a pilot study to assess recruitment and nasal sampling in newborns.

   This is a pilot study to establish if sufficient epithelial cells can be obtained from nasal samples from newborns at birth that may be used in future studies to determine gene signature patterns which may predict the development of wheeze, allergy and asthma later in childhood.
6. BENEFIT: This randomised controlled trial will investigate the effects of breastfeeding mothers eating higher dietary intakes of both egg and peanut from birth to 6 months of lactation on infant immune responses to these common food allergens. This study will inform allergy prevention recommendations.
7. CASHEW: This randomised controlled trial will investigate the effect of two different doses of regular cashew nut spread intakes during infancy on infant immune development responses to cashew nuts. The aim of this study will be to pilot regular cashew nut spread intake by infants and determine dosage recommendations prior to a larger multicentre randomised controlled trial.
8. Screen ORIGINS: First longitudinal study of the multidimensional influences and impacts of contemporary screen technology use over the first 5 years of life.

   This is an observational study, with the aim of providing a broad description of contemporary screen technology use by parents and young children, as well as to investigate associations between screen technology use and health and development outcomes. There is scarce evidence on the associations between using the newer generation of screen technology and health indicators in young children. Therefore, studies such as this are necessary to help understand how mobile screen technology use influences young children's physical and psychosocial health and development.

9. Screen ORIGINS: Qualitative investigation of parental views and practices regarding screen technology use by young children.

   This qualitative project is exploring parental views and family practices regarding screen technology use, particularly mobile technology, by young children. It is collecting data through one-on-one qualitative interviews with a subsample of parents that participate in ORIGINS. The results of this project will be valuable in informing public policy—such as public health guidelines and practice—and interventions aimed at assisting parents to promote wise use of technology by young children and future research.

A large number of other sub projects are at varying stages of development and review prior to approval by the ORIGINS executive. ORIGINS is part of a growing network of prevention intervention community cohorts aiming to improve health outcomes within an ecological framework [10]. Future sub projects nested in ORIGINS will target wellness through personalised medicine and interventions to build nature relatedness, mindfulness and positive emotions, with the aim of enhancing resilience and generating flow on effects to reduce risk targets of NCDs such as poor nutrition, physical inactivity and stress.

6.5 Input and Engagement

From the outset, the need for community engagement has been recognised to be at ORIGINS' core. There is a dedicated community stakeholder coordinator who has recruited 12 parents from the community to form the ORIGINS Community Reference Group (CRG). The CRG is actively involved in communicating community needs and assisting with the review of questionnaires, biological sampling and project plans. This group also provides guidance and informs the research questions of importance to families. In addition to the Community Reference Group, consumer and community representation is incorporated into the ORIGINS governance structure to ensure that the community is fully engaged and informed and has the opportunity to contribute meaningful input to the project. The community is represented on the ORIGINS Biobank Governance Committee; members of the CRG may attend meetings of the Scientific Committee, without voting rights; community is represented within the Translation and Health Service and Communication Services; and there is scope for a consumer representative to join the ORIGINS Executive Group in the future.

In addition to the CRG, a Participant Reference Group (PRG) was established in November 2017. All families enrolled in the project were sent an email inviting them to be part of an ongoing reference group for the project with the aim of providing feedback and guidance on the project. Ten participants indicated that they were willing to be part of the group, and four participants attended the first meeting in November 2017. The purpose of the meeting was to obtain feedback on the current practices of the project, including the recruitment process and the web-based questionnaires. It is anticipated that the PRG will provide ongoing input into the study protocol and research priorities.

Strong links have also been formed with several community and local government organisations in the surrounding, Joondalup and Wanneroo, areas. ORIGINS received endorsements from council meetings of both the City of Wanneroo and the City of Joondalup. The ORIGINS team has established strong links with the two early childhood officers at the City of Wanneroo and meet regularly to discuss ORIGINS, as well as current projects and services relating to early childhood implemented by the City of Wanneroo. This is an ongoing collaboration which has the potential to impact on policies and planning within the City of Wanneroo. Meetings have also been held with the coordinator of community development at the City of Joondalup to discuss opportunities to promote ORIGINS at local community centres, libraries, immunisation clinics and local community events within the city.

The Wanneroo and Surrounds Early Years network was established in 2004 with the aim of providing positive and improved outcomes for young children (0–8 years) and their families. Members of the ORIGINS team are members of this network and regularly attend bi-monthly meetings. These meetings are attended by representatives from a number of organisations including Ngala, Parenting Connection North West Metro, Playgroup WA, City of Wanneroo, the Smith Family, local primary schools and child care centres, as well as local government representatives. Involvement in this network has been essential in developing an understanding of the needs of the Wanneroo and Joondalup communities, as well as the existing programs and support services available to families in the area.

Ngala is a leading provider of early parenting and early childhood services for families with young children in Western Australia. Ngala is involved in a number of services in the Joondalup and Wanneroo area. This includes running the Child and Parent Centre in Neerabup, delivering parenting support in the Wanneroo/Joondalup area and running a child care facility on the JHC campus. A number of staff and families from the child care facility participated in a promotional video for ORIGINS and actively promote ORIGINS within the centre. The project links with Ngala have provided an opportunity to develop research collaborations including the development of sub projects that aim to improve antenatal and postnatal support services to new dads.

Given that general practitioners (GPs) are likely to confirm pregnancies and provide much of a woman's early antenatal care, they are an essential component of the developing community engagement and awareness of ORIGINS. In the early development of the project, the ORIGINS team visited large medical practices in the Wanneroo and Joondalup area and gave presentations about ORIGINS to the GPs. These GPs have also been given further updates regarding the progress of ORIGINS, and a workshop with a presentation on ORIGINS and the project's protocol was held at JHC. As part of the visits to the practices, the GPs were asked to complete an anonymous survey regarding a number of issues relevant to ORIGINS including current practices regarding confirmation of pregnancy, health topics discussed with pregnant patients, timing of referrals to maternity services at JHC, resources needed to discuss ORIGINS with patients and feedback on the usefulness of ORIGINS. Information obtained from the survey has been useful in developing suitable resources and materials for GPs to use to promote ORIGINS to their patients (e.g. flyers, brochures). During the discussions with GPs, it was identified that the timing of referrals to maternity services at JHC varies considerably between GPs (ranging from 8 to 36 weeks). Given that participants are required to be seen at JHC and enrolled in ORIGINS prior to 20 weeks' gestation, this would prohibit a number of women from participating in ORIGINS. As a result of this, a communication from the head of obstetrics at JHC was sent to all GP practitioners who refer antenatal patients to JHC detailing at what stage of gestation referrals should be made and outlining the appropriate paperwork and information to include in the referral documents. This has already resulted in cultural change and change in practice within the community, with stronger GP engagement, improved communication and shared care of patients and earlier referrals to the antenatal clinic at JHC by GPs. Earlier referral allows earlier detection of women with at-risk pregnancies, e.g. preeclampsia, obesity, gestational diabetes and twins. Meetings have also been held with the network support officer for the North Metropolitan division of the WA Primary Health Alliance (WAPHA). This collaboration assists in promoting ORIGINS to GPs via the WAPHA newsletter and workshops.

The Directors of ORIGINS have been in discussions with the State Government through the Chief Medical Officer, the Minister for Health and the Shadow Minister for Health. The close working relationship between the project, the community and government ensures great potential for translation into health policy and practice in WA.

A novel aspect of ORIGINS is that it is fully integrated into the clinic and diagnostic services at JHC, led by a strong cohesive vision and support of the hospital executive and all department heads. As the executive and department heads are part of the research, they drive any changes that become part of routine practice. The project crosses both public and private sectors of the Joondalup Health Campus. All departments and employees at JHC are provided with a range of opportunities to understand and become involved in ORIGINS. Clinicians, including midwives, nurses and obstetricians, have research appointments with ORIGINS in addition to their clinical duties, promoting the research culture within JHC. The ORIGINS Scientific Committee includes many leading JHC clinicians and directors. There are also a number of other JHC staff who are associate investigators on the project. This feature is an important element of the sustainability and translation plan of the project. There is international evidence that hospitals and healthcare facilities that do research deliver higher-quality care, have better patient outcomes and are more efficient [11]. A key theme in the Strategic Review of Health and Medical Research (the McKeon Review) was that the best performing health systems are those that embed research in health delivery, leading to better health outcomes [12].

In addition to the general community and clinicians, the ORIGINS Project is bringing together a large number of research collaborators to work together. All five of the WA universities (the University of Western Australia (UWA), Edith Cowan University (ECU), Curtin University, Murdoch University and Notre Dame University) are represented on the ORIGINS Scientific Committee and collaborate with the project. They contribute knowledge and facilities, such as analytical expertise and laboratory space, to enable metabolomics, metagenomics (microbiome sequencing), immunology, genetics and other analyses proposed for the project and sub projects. Further to this, Research Interest Groups (RIGs) have been set up to bring together scientists and individuals with expertise, interest and an understanding of cutting-edge research questions and technologies in specific research areas relevant to ORIGINS. The RIGs are established to help drive the project's scientific and research agenda and to create a collaborated and integrated platform for nested sub projects. Membership of the RIGs is open to researchers, clinicians, community members, consumers, service providers, academics and anyone with a particular interest and expertise. Currently there are 12 ORIGINS RIGs with a range of 6–30 members in each:

- Fathering.
- Mental Health and Wellbeing.
- Nutrition and Metabolism.
- Allergy, Inflammation and Immunity.
- Environment and Lifestyle.
- Fertility.
- Nature Relatedness.
- P4 Omics and Systems Biology.
- Oral Health.
- Epidemiology and Disadvantaged Populations.
- Growth and Development.
- Health Economics.

It is anticipated that the RIGs will continue to evolve according to the needs and interests of the project and collaborators.

Members of the RIGs represent a host of institutions, hospitals and universities, including Ngala, City of Wanneroo, The Fathering Project, Lions Eye Institute, Harry Perkins Institute of Medical Research, Fiona Stanley Hospital, Princess Margaret Hospital for Children, King Edward Memorial Hospital, TKI, JHC, Curtin, Notre Dame University, UWA, ECU and Murdoch University. Responsibilities of the RIGs include actively engaging in research collaborations and with the community, supporting scholarly activity, capacity building of early career researchers and students, provision of advisory support, identifying, generating and reviewing proposals for new sub projects and contributing expertise to enhance project and sub project success.

The ORIGINS Project brings together a broad range of collaborating parties and disciplines, all focused on taking a more integrated approach to improving a series of common health issues affecting the community. All of the engagement and collaborations enable the delivery of earlier and more targeted support for vulnerable children and their families, improving the overall health and wellbeing of the community.

Many NCDs share the same risk factors. By taking a more collaborative, interdisciplinary and harmonised approach, ORIGINS will not only build capacity to examine the complexity and interaction between multiple causative factors but also facilitate a more interdisciplinary and holistic perspective to disease prevention.

6.6 Translation and Feedback: A Responsive and Integrated System

The ORIGINS Project is investigating and creating new avenues for feedback and dissemination and ways to improve routine clinical care. For example, through the web-based questionnaires, milestones of the children's development are collected (e.g. first smile, holds a cup) using an internationally validated survey, Ages and Stages Questionnaire. JHC paediatricians monitor these results, and parents of children falling more than two standard deviations below the norm at any particular age are contacted, and a discussion around referral to GP or allied services is held. In addition, families have the option of attending child clinic assessments conducted by JHC paediatricians and allied support services when their child is 1, 2.5 and 5 years of age. This enables early identification of allergies, developmental disorders, such as language delay and delay in motor development, and neurodevelopmental disorders. Referral to appropriate allied and paediatric support within the WA Department of Health (WA DoH) and Child Development Centres (CDC) follows as necessary. Currently this is not routine care at JHC, which does not offer a public outpatient service. Early referral to the CDC, paediatricians and allied health services should result in earlier intervention for these high-risk children and improve their health and development and decrease their vulnerability.

As a result of the ORIGINS Project, a number of other changes have also already been incorporated into routine clinical practice at JHC. The JHC Mother's Health Questionnaire was revised to include more detailed and extensive questions and information for research purposes. A Father's Health Questionnaire was also developed and introduced at this time. These questionnaires are currently being routinely distributed and collected from both public and private JHC patients attending their first antenatal clinic appointment.

The ORIGINS Project is having an impact on the culture at JHC, developing as a research/clinical campus which encourages critical thinking within departments and looks to routine audits and clinical studies to ensure best practice guidelines are developed. There has been significant professional development and an active education program of JHC staff, not just about ORIGINS but related areas of evidence-based research, such as early-life nutrition and the prevention of allergy; weight gain in pregnancy, current guidelines and ways to talk to obese women about their weight.

As detailed earlier, stronger GP engagement, improved communication and shared care of patients are resulting in earlier referrals to the public antenatal clinic by GPs. On average women are now presenting approximately 4 weeks earlier, at 16 weeks GA, down from 20 weeks GA, which allows for earlier detection and management of women with at-risk pregnancies.

Trimester Club is a support and education group which for a number of years has been offered to all women in the private clinics birthing at JHC during their first pregnancy. The groups are facilitated by a clinical midwife and meet fortnightly from approximately 14 weeks' gestation until all the members have delivered.

Typically there are 20–40 women in each group. Trimester Club provides pregnant women with a friendly and nonthreatening environment where they can receive support, education and friendship through their pregnancy. The content of the group sessions is flexible but covers common themes such as common complaints in pregnancy, healthy eating and nutrition, complimentary therapies, labour process and birth, caesarean section, breastfeeding and coping after birth/postnatal depression. Informal feedback provided to the midwife who facilitates the groups indicated that these groups are valuable to the women and are important in assisting the women through their journey to becoming a mother. However, no formal feedback or evaluation of the program had ever been conducted. The ORIGINS Community Stakeholder Coordinator therefore sought and received ethical approval to obtain formal feedback from women attending Trimester Club via an anonymous questionnaire completed during the final group session. The respondents rated their experience being a part of Trimester Club during pregnancy as *Excellent* and recommended.

With the sub projects nested within the main observational cohort, any evidence-based findings from these studies that are able to reduce the risk of NCDs will have clinical translation at JHC and within the community, in conjunction with the WA Department of Health. Social media, video links on the ORIGINS Project website and news items in community newspapers will provide information on results of sub projects with education messages, e.g. breast feeding, outside play, nutrition, electronic use, etc. Further to this, ORIGINS Project families will also receive education and updates on healthy lifestyles for young children and parents via emails and newsletters. This may result in a number of positive health outcomes, e.g. improving immunisation rates and reducing obesity.

6.7 Conclusion

The health of humans, the environment, our social fabric and economic health are interconnected and interdependent. Although ORIGINS is focused specifically on health, it is really about a better future—not just locally but by contributing to global knowledge, attitudes and behaviour. We aim to bring greater awareness of the critical importance of improving conditions in early life for long-term health and longevity.

In addition to specific short-term outcomes, a large focus of ORIGINS is on promoting health and disease prevention, with a focus on healthy lifestyle, healthy food and a healthy relationship with nature and the environment. This will encourage long-range thinking and advocate strategies that might not necessarily have immediate impact, but have long-term benefits for individuals and the community into the next generations [13, 14]. For example, improving our environment in early life can benefit all aspects of our long-term physical and mental health. Moreover, it will improve health and longevity of our children.

We anticipate that the ORIGINS Project will bring people together and empower and inspire others to act and to find opportunity and common ground—all to facilitate positive change. ORIGINS will build a collaborative mindset so we can improve the health of our own future and the next generation's in *every* regard. We believe there must be stronger focus on breaking down silos and finding common ground with more mutually beneficial cross-sectoral approaches that transcend competing interests. Messages of unity and collaboration must come from science and medicine as strongly as other sectors, and this is something that will be promoted in the ORIGINS Project. This is a community cohort with extensive community engagement and participation which encourages flow on benefits for community cohesion and purpose. We aim to create an example for tailored replication in other communities and hope ORIGINS can be part of an interconnected grassroots strategy and move towards making positive change and promoting global health.

Acknowledgement The ORIGINS Project has received core funding support from the Telethon-Perth Children's Hospital Research Fund, the Paul Ramsay Foundation and the Commonwealth Government. Substantial support has also been provided by the Joondalup Health Campus and Telethon Kids Institute.

The ORIGINS Project is only possible because of the enthusiasm and commitment of the children and parents in ORIGINS. We are grateful to all the participants, health professionals and researchers who have made the ORIGINS Project happen.

We would also like to acknowledge all the members of the ORIGINS Community Reference Group, Participant Reference Group, Executive Group, Scientific Committee, Working Group, Research Interest Groups, Hospital and Project team who have supported the development and set-up of ORIGINS.

References

1. Gluckman PD, Hanson MA, Cooper C, Thornburg KL. Effect of in utero and early-life conditions on adult health and disease. N Engl J Med. 2008;359(1):61–73. https://doi.org/10.1056/NEJMra0708473.
2. Hanson MA, Gluckman PD. Developmental origins of health and Disease – Global public health implications. Best Pract Res Clin Obstet Gynaecol. 2015;29(1):24–31. https://doi.org/10.1016/j.bpobgyn.2014.06.007.
3. Prescott SL, Allen K, Armstrong K, Collins C, Dickinson H, Gardiner K, Jacka F, Jasoni C, Moore T, Moritz KM, Muhlhausler B, Siero W, Sim K, Nanan R, Saffery R, Singh G, Vickers MH, Craig JM. The establishment of DOHaD working groups in Australia and New Zealand. J Dev Orig Health Dis. 2016;7(5):433–9. https://doi.org/10.1017/S2040174416000167.
4. Balbus JM, Barouki R, Birnbaum LS, Etzel RA, Gluckman PD Sr, Grandjean P, Hancock C, Hanson MA, Heindel JJ, Hoffman K, Jensen GK, Keeling A, Neira M, Rabadan-Diehl C, Ralston J, Tang KC. Early-life prevention of non-communicable diseases. Lancet. 2013;381(9860):3–4. https://doi.org/10.1016/S0140-6736(12)61609-2.
5. Hanson M, Gluckman P, Nutbeam D, Hearn J. Priority actions for the non-communicable disease crisis. Lancet. 2011;378(9791):566–7. https://doi.org/10.1016/S0140-6736(11)61286-5.
6. President of the General Assembly. Political declaration of the High-level Meeting of the General Assembly on the Prevention and Control of Non-communicable Diseases. New York: United Nations; 2011.

7. Prescott SL. Early-life environmental determinants of allergic diseases and the wider pandemic of inflammatory noncommunicable diseases. J Allergy Clin Immunol. 2013;131(1): 23–30. https://doi.org/10.1016/j.jaci.2012.11.019.
8. Walport M, Brest P. Sharing research data to improve public health. Lancet. 2011;377(9765): 537–9. https://doi.org/10.1016/S0140-6736(10)62234-9.
9. The National Health and Medical Research Council, the Australian Research Council and the Australian Vice-Chancellors' Committee (2007) National Statement on Ethical Conduct in Human Research 2007 (Updated May 2015). Canberra: Commonwealth of Australia.
10. Prescott SL, Wegienka G, Logan AC, Katz DL. Dysbiotic drift and biopsychosocial medicine: how the microbiome links personal, public and planetary health. Biopsychosoc Med. 2018;12(7) https://doi.org/10.1186/s13030-018-0126-z.
11. National Health and Hospitals Reform Commission (2009) A healthier future for all Australians – final report of the National Health and Hospitals Reform Commission – June 2009. Canberra.
12. McKeon S, Alexander EA, Brodaty H, Ferris B, Frazer I, Little M. Strategic review of health and medical research: final report February 2013. Canberra: Australian Government Department of Health and Ageing; 2013.
13. Dubos R, Savage D, Schaedler R. Lasting effects of early environmental influences. Int J Epidemiol. 2005;34(1):5–12. https://doi.org/10.1093/ije/dyh309.
14. Prescott S, Logan A. Transforming life: a broad view of the developmental origins of health and disease concept from an ecological justice perspective. Int J Environ Res Public Health. 2016;13(11):1075.

Chapter 7
Growing Up in New Zealand: A Prebirth Cohort Study of Child Wellbeing and Development

Susan M. B. Morton

Abstract *Growing Up in New Zealand* is the contemporary prebirth longitudinal cohort study established to understand what shapes developmental trajectories for the current generation of New Zealand children in the context of their diverse families and broader social environments. The study provides population-relevant evidence relevant to the Developmental Origins of Health and Adult Disease paradigm by collecting detailed social and biological information to understand what shapes early development to understand what works to give every child the best possible start to life.

The cohort of 6853 children engaged in the *Growing Up in New Zealand* longitudinal study from before their birth are broadly generalisable to all contemporary births in New Zealand. Of particular importance is that the cohort of children represent the ethnic diversity of the current generation of New Zealand children and the socio-demographic characteristics of their diverse families.

From the development phase onwards, *Growing Up in New Zealand* has created partnerships with policymakers across multiple government sectors to facilitate the collection of relevant information and enable the timely translation of the research findings. Policy relevance and utility is a key goal for *Growing Up in New Zealand*, and to date the evidence from the cohort has informed policies in the perinatal period in areas such as maternity care, breastfeeding, immunisation and parental leave and return to work in the postnatal period.

Keywords Longitudinal study · Birth cohort · Recruitment and retention · Child health and wellbeing · Developmental trajectories · Life course epidemiology · Policy translation

---

S. M. B. Morton
University of Auckland, Auckland, New Zealand
e-mail: s.morton@auckland.ac.nz

F. Sata et al. (eds.), *Pre-emptive Medicine: Public Health Aspects of Developmental Origins of Health and Disease*, Current Topics in Environmental Health and Preventive Medicine, https://doi.org/10.1007/978-981-13-2194-8_7

Abbreviations

CAPI	Computer-assisted personal interview
CATI	Computer-assisted telephone interview
DCW	Data collection wave
DOHAD	Developmental Origins of Health and Disease
GUINZ	Growing Up in New Zealand
NZ	New Zealand

7.1 Introduction

Growing Up in New Zealand is a longitudinal, multi-disciplinary prebirth cohort study designed specifically to understand what shapes developmental trajectories for contemporary New Zealand children growing up in the context of their diverse families in dynamic interaction with their multiple environments in the twenty-first century. The study's explicit objective is to be translational; that is, to provide population-relevant evidence about what influences children's wellbeing, to inform the evaluation and implementation of cross-sectorial policy initiatives that can improve the health and wellbeing of all New Zealand children. In terms of application to the Developmental Origins of Health and Disease, the study has specifically focussed on collecting detailed information to understand what shapes development in the critical first thousand days of children's lives to understand what works best to optimise the wellbeing for all children and to give everyone the best possible start to life.

7.2 Research Design

The conceptual framework for *Growing Up in New Zealand* is based on a life course epidemiological framework. Such a framework considers influences on development through multiple contexts and how proximal and distal influences accumulate, overlap and also change over time to impact wellbeing [1–4].

The 6853 children in the *Growing Up in New Zealand* cohort are central to all data collections, but the conceptual framework recognizes that they only develop in dynamic interaction with their families, communities and wider physical environments and societal contexts over time. This conceptual approach acknowledges the growth in understanding of early child development in the last few decades, including the emergence of the Developmental Origins of Health and Disease (DOHAD) paradigm, with the increasing recognition in particular of the importance of the first thousand days of life, including the antenatal and pre-pregnancy periods, for setting developmental pathways that will potentially shape outcomes into adulthood.

The model therefore incorporates the notion that the development of all children begins from before they are born (intergenerational continuity) as well as the notion

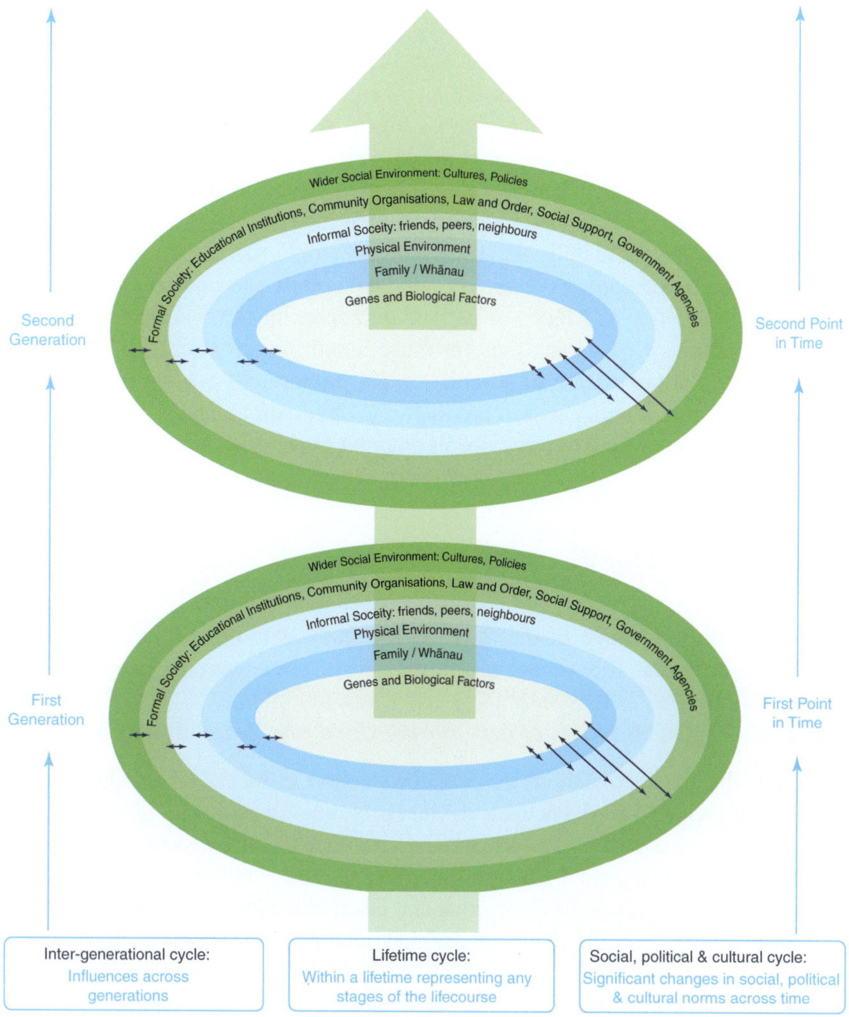

Fig. 7.1 Conceptual framework of Growing Up in New Zealand

that each life course outcome is the result of a complex interplay between the individual's biology and their proximal and distal environments over time [5] (Fig. 7.1).

In particular the *Growing Up in New Zealand* study:

- Describes antenatal and intergenerational influences on child development (recruiting in pregnancy and beginning data collection before birth).
- Emphasises the importance of early life data (in particular the first thousand days of development).
- Includes data collected independently from fathers (and partners) from before birth.
- Takes an interdisciplinary and life course approach to child development.

7.3 Cohort Description

The cohort of children engaged in the *Growing Up in New Zealand* longitudinal study is generalizable to all contemporary births in New Zealand according to the key demographic characteristics of child ethnicity, parental markers of socioeconomic status and urban/rural residential mix. A cost-efficient, geographical sampling frame is used to recruit the children via their mothers and mother's partners in pregnancy [6]. The postnatally determined final sample size of 6853 children provides adequate explanatory power to undertake robust life course analyses with children who identify as Māori, in particular (approximately one in four of New Zealand births), as well as analyses for those identifying as Pacific and Asian, as well as across the population of all children [7]. Importantly a large proportion of the cohort children identify with more than one ethnic group and ethnic identity is likely to change over time as other developmental trajectories also evolve.

7.4 Research Questions

The overarching objective of the longitudinal study is to determine what factors shape developmental life course trajectories for a contemporary cohort of New Zealand children, as well as within key subgroups of children.

Specifically, the objectives of the *Growing Up in New Zealand* study are:

- To map the developmental trajectories for a cohort of New Zealand children as a group, and within Māori, Pacific and Asian subgroups in particular, in order to identify the main causal pathways, and the links between them, across multiple levels of influence (political, social, cultural, intergenerational, familial and individual) for outcomes in key social, developmental and health domains across the life course.
- To provide a description of cross-sectional outcomes (in several domains) at key points in the life course of the developing child and to enable comparisons between and within subgroups and against international populations.
- To focus on factors and trajectories, across multiple levels of influence, that confer resilience and optimise development, rather than focusing solely on risk factors for poor outcomes.
- To identify critical or sensitive periods in development, and levels of influence, that will inform policies directed at optimising the development of every child born in New Zealand.

7.5 Data Collection Waves (2008–2016)

Trajectories of early life development from before birth are recognised as critical for influencing the ongoing health, wellbeing and resilience of children and their families in the DOHAD paradigm as well as in life course epidemiology. Accordingly five significant data collection waves have been conducted within the first 5 years of the children's lives to provide detailed information about the children's early development. Each data collection wave of *Growing Up in New Zealand* seeks age-appropriate information across the six interconnected domains: family and whānau; neighbourhood, environment and societal context; education; health and wellbeing; psychological and cognitive development; and culture and identity. Methods to collect domain-specific evidence acknowledge the unique New Zealand population and environmental context, particularly the unique opportunity *Growing Up in New Zealand* has to examine the factors which contribute to the wellbeing of Māori whānau in New Zealand in the twenty-first century.

Traditional methods of computer-assisted telephone interviews (CATI) and computer-assisted personal interviews (CAPI) have been augmented by linkage to information from routine datasets throughout the early data collection waves. In addition, electronic and text contact, incentives, competitions and the use of social media support information gathering. The longitudinal information collected to date (up to December 2016), using multiple methods, includes the following.

7.5.1 *Face-to-Face Interviews*

Face-to-face interviews conducted as computer-assisted personal interviews (CAPI) have been utilised for:

- The antenatal data collection wave (DCW) in 2009–2010 with the pregnant mother (most often in the last trimester of her pregnancy) and with her partner (almost always the biological father).
- The 9-month DCW with the child's mother and her partner (2010–2011).
- The 2-year DCW with the child's mother and her partner (2011–2012), which also involved direct observations and developmental and anthropometric assessments of the children at 2 years of age.
- The 4-year DCW with the child's mother (completed in 2014–2015), which also involved direct observations and developmental and anthropometric assessments of the children at 4.5 years of age.

7.5.2 *Telephone Interviews*

Telephone interviews are conducted as computer-assisted telephone interviews (CATI).

- These occurred when the children were aged approximately 6 weeks, 35 weeks, 16 months, 23 months, 31 months and 45 months.

The telephone interviews provide valuable, age-appropriate information that enhances the data collected face-to-face.

7.5.3 Data Linkage

- Linkage between the *Growing Up in New Zealand* data and routinely collected perinatal health records was undertaken in 2012.
- Parental consent for linkage to routine education and health data up to the age of 7 years was obtained at the 4-year face-to-face interview.

All questionnaires used in the field are made available on the *Growing Up in New Zealand* website (www.growingup.co.nz) once a data wave collection is completed in the field. Biological samples were obtained from the children around the time of birth (dried blood spots) and also at the preschool interview (saliva samples for DNA extraction and bacterial swabs for colonisation information).

The data collection mode and timing is summarised in Table 7.1.

A summary of the information collected is provided in Table 7.2. Longitudinal information is collected to provide measures of child development as well as proximal and distal broader familial, societal and environmental influences. Information is collected to inform trajectory development rather than cross-sectional status per se, and collection of information is only repeated when sufficient change is expected to have occurred at the population level to justify this.

Cohort retention rates have remained very high compared with similar international cohort studies and compared to predicted rates when the study was designed. Less than 4% of the baseline cohort have opted out of the longitudinal study altogether over the first five data collection waves. Rates of completion of each data collection wave are slightly lower than this, however, given that some families skip a particular collection wave but still agree to remain in the cohort for future contact and data collection.

For example, information was collected for over 90% of cohort (6156 children) at the 54-month or 4-year data collection point (7% skips). This high retention rate has occurred in the face of great residential mobility of the families, half of whom

Table 7.1 Data collection mode and timing

Child age	Antenatal	Perinatal	< 9 months	9 months	< 2 years	2 years	< 4 years	4.5 years
CAPI[a]	✓			✓		✓		✓
CATI[b]			✓		✓		✓	
Child[c]		✓				✓		✓
Data linkage		✓	✓	✓	✓	✓	✓	✓
Bio sample[d]		✓						✓

[a]CAPI computer-assisted personal interview
[b]CATI computer-assisted telephone interview
[c]Child measurement
[d]Saliva samples, throat/nasal/skin swabs, dried blood spots, cord blood (subsample)

Table 7.2 Summary of overarching constructs measured throughout *Growing Up in New Zealand*

Child characteristics	Distal social environments
• Early life injuries • Size at birth and perinatal health • Child anthropometry • Psychosocial and cognitive development • Behaviour and temperament	• Neighbourhood (physical location, integration, access to services, informal support available) • Transport and access to local services • Early childhood education • Well child checks • Interaction with social services
Proximal social environments	**Macro environmental factors**
• Family structure, including parents, siblings and extended family • Child's home physical and social environment • Parental physical and mental health • Household deprivation • Parental stress and support • Parent-child interaction • Ethnic identity • Safety practices in the home	• Continuity of access to primary health care services • Healthcare cost • Parental labour force status • Early childhood education • Family support measures including any family taxation relief or benefits • Housing tenure • Residential mobility

have moved between each data collection wave. Of the 6156 children with completed interviews at the age of 4 years, 4165 (68%) were identified as NZ European, 1522 (25%) as Māori, 1263 (21%) as Pacific and 1027(16%) as Asian, with multiple ethnicities identified for nearly half of the cohort. Attrition bias has been minimal with respect to key parameters of ethnicity and socioeconomic status (see Fig. 7.2). Biological samples were obtained from the cohort at 4 years of age [8], saliva samples for genetic analyses were collected from 4975 (81%) and consent for linkage to healthcare data obtained for 5637(92%) of the children.

7.6 Utilising the Longitudinal Information

Longitudinal data collected to date from the children and their families provide information regarding child-specific factors, familial factors, extended family and wider social networks (the proximal social environment), informal and formal supports (the distal social environments) and the wider societal, cultural, economic and policy context (the macro-environmental factors) that shape contemporary New Zealand child developmental trajectories. From the development phase onwards, *Growing Up in New Zealand* has created partnerships with policymakers across multiple sectors to facilitate the relevance of and the translation of the research findings. Policy relevance and utility is a key goal for *Growing Up in New Zealand.* This is achieved through (1) specific translational objectives and research questions, (2) engagement with policymakers throughout the design phase and (3) continued and ongoing engagement with policymakers at all steps of data collection and dissemination. This engagement is mediated by the *Growing Up in New Zealand* policy

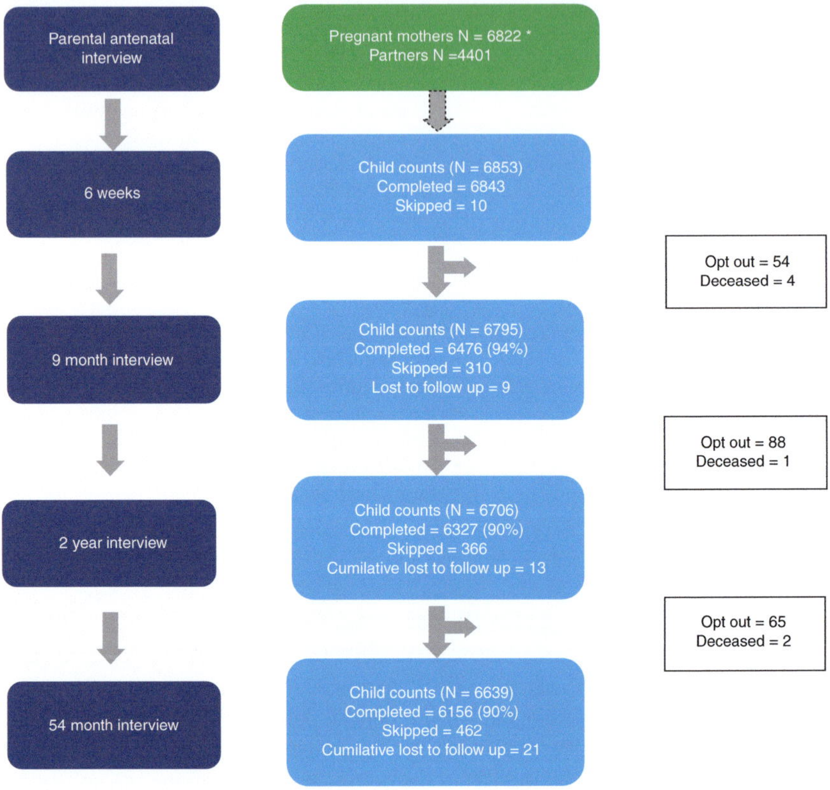

Fig. 7.2 Cohort retention rates. *Notes*. *Complete antenatal interview data (1) 'Skipped' refers to a mother unable to provide information at a specific data collection point but still intending to complete subsequent data collection waves. (2) 'Lost to follow-up' refers to a participant who could not be contacted at this specific DCW. (3) 'Opt out' refers to a participant who has specifically indicated that they no longer wish to participate in the study; where this is a mother, her participant child or children are therefore opted out. (4) Percentage of 'completed'—the denominator for completed DCWs is the total live births determined at the 6-week call ($N = 6853$)

forum, a multi-agency reference group of senior policy advisors representing the New Zealand Families Commission/Social Policy Research Evaluation Unit, Statistics New Zealand, Office of Ethnic Affairs, Te Puni Kokiri, Ministries of Health, Justice, Social Development, Women's Affairs, Pacific Island Affairs, Education and the Office of the Children's Commissioner. This forum meets several times a year to review data collection plans and data analysis and inform reporting and translation of research and policy outputs.

Analyses applied to the longitudinal information respect the temporal nature of the information and the highly correlated, repeated measures of both child development and the broader environment collected at different points in time. The advantage of having repeated measures on the same group of individuals is significant as it allows analyses to identify changes in an individual's status over time, as well as to highlight what conditions or factors have contributed to change, noting that this change may reflect either improvement or worsening of exposures or outcomes. The repeated information also allows an understanding of what factors and environments contribute to stability of exposure and chronicity of either good or poor outcomes. Applying this methodological approach means that the information from the cohort is able to inform when, how, what and for whom strategies should be optimally targeted to improve wellbeing and give every NZ child a better start to life. This repeated information on the same individuals, their families and their environmental contexts is not readily available from routine administrative datasets alone.

The longitudinal information provides a valuable and unique research resource to investigate DOHaD concepts and to inform policy and research. The longitudinal data resource was (and continues to be) designed to have utility for multiple users including researchers, policymakers and other stakeholders. It is intended to be used widely without jeopardising the privacy, confidentiality or continuing involvement of the longitudinal study participants.

Researchers external to the *Growing Up in New Zealand* team are able to apply to use anonymised datasets for bona fide research. There is a detailed and well-defined application process that involves approval for access by a Data Access Committee, which is guided by a Data Access Protocol, to ensure that external applicants and all data access requests comply with a set of strict criteria intended to protect the anonymity of participants (according to existing study ethical agreements and participant consents), and which protect the long-term sustainability of the study.

7.7 Next Steps

The longitudinal research is ongoing and is expected to continue until the children are at least 21 years of age. Planning for a data collection wave in 2017, when the children are 8 years old, is underway. The 8-year data collection will be the first face-to-face collection of information since the children entered formal schooling (after their fifth birthday in New Zealand), so it represents an important transition in their lives, a transition that will critically shape their future developmental outcomes, adult wellbeing and engagement with wider society. The 8-year data collection plans include a school module as well as mother-and-child interviews and direct observations of development and wellbeing and repeat biological sampling.

It is anticipated that data collections will continue every 2–3 years, to capture key transitions such as puberty and adolescence, transition to secondary education and then transition to advanced training, tertiary education and/or labour force participation. These regular data collections will also ensure that the early life longitudinal information will have maximal utility to inform what shapes developmental trajectories to adulthood for children growing up in New Zealand today.

7.8 Making a Difference and Demonstrating Impact

Growing Up in New Zealand has deliberately sought to use information in as timely a way as possible and has delivered a greater number of outputs in the first 5 years than historical New Zealand longitudinal studies and many contemporary international cohort studies. Given the longitudinal nature of data collections, it is also imperative that in the early years of a longitudinal study, the recruitment and the retention strategies create a robust foundation for the information that will be collected over time, and there are few shortcuts to achieve this [5, 9–13].

The rich information that has been generated from the preschool data collections has already provided a valuable resource for multiple researchers to investigate key research questions relating to early life development and potential risks or protective factors for later life health and wellbeing. For example, by the time the children enter formal schooling, they are 'digital natives', and the environments they are growing up in are vastly different from those of the previous generations in New Zealand. The cohort children are less likely to live in a nuclear family (69%) and more likely to be living in an extended family environment (20%) than with only one parent (5%). Their families are highly mobile (one in four moved in their first year of life, a further one in three before their second birthday and one in two again before they were 5 years old). Only half are living in homes that their families own. Their mothers are more likely to be working than were mothers in previous generations, but families with young children are still more likely to be experiencing greater hardship in terms of material deprivation than other New Zealanders. The children are also likely to be multilingual, with one in three having at least one parent who was not born in New Zealand. Obesity is common in the cohort with almost 15% overweight or obese by the time they enter primary school (up from 10% when they are 2 years old). Obesity is already more common in Maori and Pacific children than in NZ European or Asian groups, although no groups are immune. A genetic variant (CREBRF) has also been identified within the cohort, most commonly in Māori and Pacific children, that is not related to birth weight but which is related to differential postnatal growth rates and could represent a different response in these children to the same environments.

The rich longitudinal information from the families has provided evidence to inform policy change including the recent changes to New Zealand's paid parental leave policy and to the introduction of the 'Warrant of Fitness' for rental properties, given the high proportion of young children who now grow up in families apparently destined to be lifelong renters (almost half of the cohort). Information has also been provided to inform early identification of children who are most vulnerable to adversity and early life poor outcomes from the time of their birth. This has led to suggestions about how to more accurately target the way health-related services are provided to the most vulnerable families from the perinatal period (before their children are born), to avoid downstream issues before they arise and optimise these children's start to life. Importantly, the longitudinal information collected directly from the families and children provides opportunities to identify factors that create resilience in the face of adversity for the most vulnerable children [14]; in other words, to identify what *is* working for children and families in contemporary New Zealand society and how we can apply this to ensure all New Zealand children have the opportunity to thrive and flourish. (All outputs can be viewed at the study website: www.growingup.co.nz.)

7.9 Conclusion

Growing Up in New Zealand continues to collect multidisciplinary information to determine what influences early development for contemporary New Zealand children, and how early life characteristics are related to wellbeing and development in later life. The intent is to ensure that this longitudinal evidence informs cross-sectoral strategies to improve the health and wellbeing of all future New Zealanders. The voices of the children themselves are now adding value to the collection of information as they move into early adolescence. Every child in the cohort has a unique story to tell, and each contributes to the collection of rich longitudinal information over time. By following the lives of these ordinary New Zealand children and their families, and telling their stories, there is a real opportunity to make an extraordinary difference for all New Zealand children and inform population relevant ways to give every child the best possible early start to life and therefore the best chance of a healthy life course.

Appendix: Domain-Specific Research Questions for Growing Up in New Zealand

1. What are the developmental pathways that determine the health status of children across the life course from antenatal development to early adulthood?
2. How does an individual's biological profile, and the environment in which they grow, mutually interact over time to influence development?
3. What are the key determinants of the developmental trajectories that lead to behavioural, emotional and social competence in childhood and adolescence, and what precipitates either continuity or change in these trajectories?
4. What biological and environmental factors impact on cognitive ability, and how do these factors influence developmental outcomes and trajectories over the life course?
5. How do the multiple levels of self, family, environment and educational context and composition influence and affect educational and developmental outcomes over time?
6. What factors influence academic motivation, perceived academic competence and educational achievement across the life course, in particular at key transition points?

7. How does the quality of family/whānau dynamics including sibling, parent-child, inter-parental and relationships with extended family influence children's development over time?
8. How do children's experiences of family/whānau life vary, and what factors confer resilience or present risks to their development, in diverse family forms and during periods of family transition?
9. How involved are fathers in children's lives, and what are their influences over time on children's development?
10. How are culture and ethnic identity understood and 'shaped' for children and their families, and what developmental trajectories are associated with cross-cultural parental and child ethnicities across the life course?
11. What influences do the physical, social and cultural environments have on children and their families' cultural experiences and identities in terms of holistic development?
12. What are the key features (social networks, infrastructure and physical environment) of neighbourhoods and communities which impact on an individual's development over time?
13. What role do neighbourhoods and communities have in mediating the associations between family circumstances, dynamics and social conditions (SES) and child development? How does geographic mobility influence this effect?
14. How important is engagement of the family and child with key social services and institutions—including health, education and social service providers—in affecting child outcomes? What factors in the social and family environment facilitate effective engagement?
15. How are diverse social and economic contexts expressed in family values, practices, beliefs and resources? How are child outcomes shaped by the effect of these social contexts on family values, practices, beliefs and resources?
16. How are child outcomes affected by the nature of their parents' workforce participation, and what factors both internal and external to the family modify these effects?
17. What effects do mass media, communications and new technologies have on children's health and development, and what factors in the family and social environment modify these effects?
18. How do New Zealand policies affect the social and economic positioning of the cohort families/whānau, what stressors or enablers do they create and how do they impact on child development?

References

1. Ben-Shlomo Y, Kuh D. A life course approach to chronic disease epidemiology: conceptual models, empirical challenges, and interdisciplinary perspectives. Int J Epidemiol. 2002;31:285–93.
2. Bronfenbrenner U. The ecology of human development: experiments by nature and design. Cambridge, MA: Harvard University Press; 1979.

3. Dahlgren G, Whitehead M. Policies and strategies to promote social equity in health. Stockholm: Institute for Futures Studies; 1991.
4. Lynch J, Smith GD. A life course approach to chronic disease epidemiology. Annu Rev Public Health. 2005;26:1–35.
5. Morton SM, Atatoa Carr PE, Grant CC, Robinson EM, Bandara DK, Bird A, et al. Cohort profile: Growing Up in New Zealand. Int J Epidemiol. 2012a;42:65–75. https://doi.org/10.1093/ije/dyr206.
6. Poulton R, Hancox R, Milne B, Baxter J, Scott K, Wilson N. The Dunedin Multidisciplinary Health and Development Study: are its findings consistent with the overall New Zealand population? N Z Med J. 2006;119(1235):U2002.
7. Shulruf B, Morton SM, Goodyear-Smith F, O'Loughlin C, Dixon R. Designing multidisciplinary longitudinal studies of human development analyzing past research to inform methodology. Eval Health Prof. 2007;30(3):207–28.
8. Berry S, Morton S, Atatoa Carr P, et al. Colonisation with Staphylococcus aureus and Streptococcus pyogenes in New Zealand preschool children. N Z Med J. 2015;128(1410):60–7.
9. Morton S, Atatoa Carr PE, Bandara DK, et al. Growing Up in New Zealand: A longitudinal study of New Zealand children and their families. Report 1: before we are born. Auckland, NZ: University of Auckland; 2010.
10. Morton SMB, Grant CC, Atatoa Carr PE, Robinson EM, Kinloch JM, Fleming CJ, Kingi TKR, Perese LM, Liang R. How do you recruit and retain a pre-birth cohort? Lessons learnt from Growing Up in New Zealand. Eval Health Prof. 2012b;37(4):411–33. https://doi.org/10.1177/0163278712462717.
11. Morton SM, Atatoa Carr P, Grant CC, et al. Growing Up in New Zealand: A longitudinal study of New Zealand children and their families. Now we are two: describing our first 1000 days. Auckland, NZ: Growing Up in New Zealand; 2014a.
12. Morton SMB, Atatoa Carr PE, Grant CC, et al. Growing Up in New Zealand: A longitudinal study of New Zealand children and their families. Vulnerability Report 1: Exploring the definition of vulnerability for children in their first 1000 days. Auckland, NZ: Growing Up in New Zealand; 2014b.
13. Morton SMB, Atatoa Carr PE, Berry S, Grant CC. Growing Up in New Zealand: A longitudinal study of New Zealand children and their families. Mobility Report 1: residential mobility in their first 1000 days. Auckland, NZ: Growing Up in New Zealand; 2014c.
14. Morton, S.M., Berry, S.D., Atatoa Carr, P.E., Grant, C.C., & Pillai, A. (2015b). Growing Up in New Zealand Vulnerability Report 2: transitions in exposure to vulnerability in the first 1000 days of life. Commissioning body: Superu.

Chapter 8
Public Health Aspect of the Growing Up in Singapore Towards Healthy Outcomes (GUSTO) Mother-Offspring Cohort

Shu-E Soh, Fabian Yap, Kok Hian Tan, Lynette Pei-Chi Shek, Keith M. Godfrey, Michael J. Meaney, Peter D. Gluckman, and Yap-Seng Chong

S.-E. Soh
Singapore Institute for Clinical Sciences, Agency for Science, Technology and Research, Singapore, Singapore

Department of Paediatrics, Yong Loo Lin School of Medicine, National University of Singapore, Singapore, Singapore
e-mail: Soh_Shu_E@sics.a-star.edu.sg

F. Yap · K. H. Tan
KK Women's and Children's Hospital, Singapore, Singapore
e-mail: fabian.yap.k.p@singhealth.com.sg; tan.kok.hian@singhealth.com.sg

L. P.-C. Shek
Department of Paediatrics, Yong Loo Lin School of Medicine, National University of Singapore, Singapore, Singapore
e-mail: paeshekl@nus.edu.sg

K. M. Godfrey
MRC Lifecourse Epidemiology Unit and NIHR Southampton Biomedical Research Centre, University of Southampton and University Hospital Southampton NHS Foundation Trust, Southampton, UK
e-mail: kmg@mrc.soton.ac.uk

M. J. Meaney
Singapore Institute for Clinical Sciences, Agency for Science, Technology and Research, Singapore, Singapore

McGill University, Montreal, QC, Canada
e-mail: michael.meaney@mcgill.ca

P. D. Gluckman
Singapore Institute for Clinical Sciences, Agency for Science, Technology and Research, Singapore, Singapore

Liggins Institute, University of Auckland, Auckland, New Zealand
e-mail: pd.gluckman@auckland.ac.nz

F. Sata et al. (eds.), *Pre-emptive Medicine: Public Health Aspects of Developmental Origins of Health and Disease*, Current Topics in Environmental Health and Preventive Medicine, https://doi.org/10.1007/978-981-13-2194-8_8

Y.-S. Chong (✉)
Singapore Institute for Clinical Sciences, Agency for Science, Technology and Research, Singapore, Singapore

Department of Obstetrics and Gynaecology, Yong Loo Lin School of Medicine, National University of Singapore, Singapore, Singapore
e-mail: obgcys@nus.edu.sg, yap_seng_chong@sics.a-star.edu.sg

Abstract The Growing Up in Singapore Towards Healthy Outcomes (GUSTO) cohort study was established in 2009 and recruited 1247 Chinese, Malay, and Indian families to precisely define the critical developmental pathways and mechanisms of the origins of obesity, metabolic disease, and neurodevelopmental disorders that have major public health and economic importance in Asia and globally, with the goal to develop precision medicine approaches (biomarkers and interventions) for families at risk of future noncommunicable diseases. Our studies have already had major academic and translational impact and attracted significant media attention and policymakers' interest. Some examples of the translation of our science into public health activities are in the area of gestational diabetes mellitus, maternal emotional well-being, and preconception and antenatal nutritional intervention to develop better nutrition guidelines for prospective parents, pregnant women, infants, and children.

Keywords Metabolic disease · Neurodevelopment · Asia · Precision medicine · Health policy

Abbreviations

25OHD	Serum 25-hydroxyvitamin D
ADHD	Attention deficit hyperactivity disorder
BMI	Body mass index
CI	Confidence interval
COMT	catechol-*O*-methyltransferase
DOHaD	Developmental Origins of Health and Disease
EDPS	Edinburgh Postnatal Depression Scale
GDM	Gestational diabetes mellitus
GUSTO	Growing Up in Singapore Towards Healthy Outcomes
GxE	Gene-environment interactions
KKH	KK Women's and Children's Hospital, Singapore
MRI	Magnetic resonance imaging
NCD	Noncommunicable disease
NUH	National University Hospital, Singapore
SD	Standard deviation
STAI	Spielberger State-Trait Anxiety Inventory

8.1 Introduction

The Growing Up in Singapore Towards Healthy Outcomes (GUSTO) study is a deeply phenotyped mother-offspring cohort designed to address hypotheses that are core to the DOHaD paradigm. The emerging epidemic and evolution of noncommunicable diseases (NCDs), including obesity, metabolic disease, and neurodevelopmental disorders, in developed and developing countries, has become one of the greatest public health challenges of the twenty-first century [1, 2].

Southeast Asia has the second largest population of diabetics in the world, with an estimated regional prevalence of 8.5% in 2015, projected to grow to 10.7% by 2040 [3]. In Singapore, the prevalence of type 2 diabetes mellitus has increased more than fivefold in the last four decades [4]; the International Diabetes Foundation estimated the national prevalence of diabetes (aged 20–79) for Singapore to be 12.8% in 2015 [3], now one of the highest in the developed world. A complex interplay of gene-environment interactions (GxE) underlies the early developmental pathways leading to obesity, insulin resistance, and eventual metabolic disease later on in life [5, 6]. South Asians, albeit having lower body mass index (BMI) than Caucasians, generally are more prone to central adiposity and more likely to be diagnosed with metabolic diseases such as type 2 diabetes [7, 8]. The GUSTO mother-offspring cohort presents a unique opportunity to study ethnic differences among three populous Asian ethnicities that appear to have distinct susceptibilities, leading to differing metabolic risk, the Chinese, Malay, and Indian, who together comprise over 50% of the global population.

In addition to investigating the developmental precursors to metabolic compromise leading to obesity, diabetes, and cardiovascular morbidity, GUSTO further aims to understand the precursors of the cognitive and emotional abilities that define mental health and human capital across the life span. Analysis of epidemiological datasets suggests that early developmental pathways that render individuals vulnerable for psychopathology involve parental mental health and family quality and that these influences are moderated by child genotype and mediated by epigenetic mechanisms [9]. The GUSTO cohort represents a remarkable opportunity for the study of comorbid health conditions. We focus especially on comorbid metabolic, inflammatory, and mental health conditions.

Our research objectives are to more precisely define the critical developmental pathways and mechanisms of the origins of obesity, metabolic disease, and neurodevelopmental disorders that have major public health and economic importance in Asia and globally, with the goal of developing precision medicine approaches (biomarkers and interventions) for children at risk of future NCDs. Precision interventions will require the integration of clinically relevant environmental conditions with information on the child's genotype and additional potential moderators (e.g., epigenetic).

The science that we are studying is still relatively unexplored (featured by TIME magazine to be a new field in October 2010) [10] and will provide incredible opportunities to discover and develop new strategies to promote population health and enhance human capacity.

8.2 Methods and Protocol

The GUSTO mother-offspring cohort was established in 2009 and recruited 1247 Chinese, Malay, and Indian pregnant women who were of homogenous parental ethnic background in their first trimester from the two major public maternity hospitals in Singapore, National University Hospital (NUH) and KK Women's and Children's Hospital (KKH) [11]. There were four detailed ultrasound scans at 11–12, 19–21, 26–28, and 32–34 weeks' gestation, with in-depth phenotyping at recruitment and 26–28 weeks' gestation to capture data on demography, socioeconomic status, lifestyle, maternal emotional well-being, obstetric and medical history, dietary patterns, and cardio-metabolic status. An oral glucose tolerance test was conducted at 26–28 weeks of gestation with analyses of other biochemical markers.

After delivery, the children have been closely followed up and deeply phenotyped and are now about 8–9 years old (retention rate: 82%). They have undergone in-depth auxological, cardio-metabolic, and neuropsychiatric assessments since birth, with 3-monthly follow-up until 15 months of age and thereafter every 6 months from 18 months to 8 years of age. A subset had whole-body magnetic resonance imaging (MRI) for brain and body composition and detailed neurodevelopmental assessments in early childhood.

Biospecimens collected include maternal blood, umbilical cord, cord blood and placenta at delivery, serial buccal swabs, breastmilk, hair, and fecal samples from the parents and child (Fig. 8.1). As one of the most deeply and closely phenotyped and biosampled birth cohorts in the world, we will exploit our strength and extensive capacity in systems biology with our EpiGen consortium collaborators in Auckland, New Zealand, and Southampton, United Kingdom, to perform sophisticated analyses of genotype, epigenotype-developmental, and environment-phenotype relationships as the children grow and develop. This will allow us to develop evidence-based "precision prevention" strategy that identifies the impact of environmental adversity at the level of the individual child. These same analyses will allow us to examine epigenetic marks that reflect gene-environment interactions, as specific biomarkers of vulnerability.

As the children in GUSTO enter formal school age (from 6 years) and puberty (from 9 years), our ability to extend cohort phenotyping (e.g., blood sampling of the children) and study more meaningful neurodevelopmental, metabolic, and endocrine outcomes will further increase the scientific and public health impact of the program.

8.3 Public Health Recommendations

Understanding the biology of developmental programming of NCDs and its translation into advances in prevention and intervention strategies targeting healthy childhood development and reducing the risk of metabolic and mental diseases has the potential for substantial impact on the current public policy and health service

Measures	Pregnancy	Delivery	Postnatal																		
	4 visits		Week 3	6	Month 3	6	9	12	15	18	Year 2	3	3.5	4	4.5	5	5.5	6	6.5	7	8
Mother																					
Demographic and lifestyle data	x																	x			x
Physical and mental health	x				x	x		x		x	x		x	x	x			x			x
Obstetric data	x	x																			
Diet and nutrition	x		x		x	x		x										x			
Physical examination	x					x				x				x				x			x
Biological samples collected	x	x	x		x	x								x				x			x
Father																					
Demographic and lifestyle data	x										x	x									
Physical health			x								x	x			x						
Physical examination											x	x									
Biological samples collected											x	x			x	x					
Infant/Child																					
Growth & Body Composition	x	x	x	x	x	x	x	x	x	x	x	x		x	x	x	x	x	x	x	x
Diet and Nutrition			x		x	x	x	x	x	x	x	x		x		x		x	x	x	
Food preference & eating behaviour					x			x	x			x				x		x		x	
Illnesses & Allergies			x		x	x	x	x	x	x	x	x		x		x		x		x	x
Cognitive function		x		x	x	x	x	x		x	x		x	x	x			x		x	
Magnetic resonance imaging (MRI)		x		x		x									x	x		x		x	
Developmental milestones/language						x	x	x		x	x		x	x	x			x			
Social Emotional Assessment					x	x	x	x		x	x		x		x			x			
Executive functioning											x		x	x	x			x			
Sleep/physical activity						x		x		x	x		x		x		x				x
School readiness														x							
Dental eruption & Oral health						x	x	x	x	x	x	x		x		x		x			
Eye assessment												x						x			
Pubertal assessment																		x		x	x
Cardiovascular assessment																		x			
Environmental exposure						x		x				x				x	x	x			x
Health expenditure									x	x	x	x				x					
Biological samples collected																					
Buccal swab		x	x		x	x	x	x	x	x	x	x	x	x	x	x	x	x	x	x	x
Nasal swab			x		x	x	x	x	x	x											
Stools		x	x		x	x		x			x			x							x
Hair														x	x			x		x	x
Blood																		x			x
Urine																				x	x
Exfoliated teeth																		x			

Fig. 8.1 Information collected by questionnaires, physical measurements and biological samples in the GUSTO cohort study

practices in Asia and globally. Our studies have already had major academic and translational impact and attracted significant media attention [12–15] and policy-makers' interest [16–19]. Some examples of the translation of our science into action are highlighted here.

8.3.1 Gestational Diabetes Mellitus

In Singapore, gestational diabetes mellitus (GDM) is much more prevalent than previously thought, affecting up to one in five women, with differing frequency for Chinese, Malay, and Indian women [20]. The high-risk approach previously recommended by local authorities for screening women for GDM misses half the actual cases (Table 8.1).

We found that even in the absence of GDM, higher fasting glucose levels can affect infant adiposity and neural development, suggesting that medical observation and evaluation are needed at levels below the formal diagnostic criteria. Each standard deviation (SD) increase in fasting glucose was associated with 31% [95% confidence interval (CI) 1.10–1.55], 72% (95% CI 1.31–2.27), and 64%

Table 8.1 Proportion of detected gestational diabetes mellitus (GDM) in GUSTO cohort using universal versus high-risk screening[a] (Modified from [20])

Screening method	Whole cohort (n = 1135)	Chinese (n = 646)	Malay (n = 286)	Indian (n = 203)
Universal[b]	218 (19.2)	137 (21.2)	32 (11.2)	49 (24.1)
High risk[b]	121 (10.7)[c]	58 (9.0)[c]	28 (9.8)[c]	35 (17.2)[c]

[a]Values are given as number (%)
[b]Universal screening is where all participants undergo oral glucose tolerance test (OGTT); high-risk screening is where only participants with one or more of the risk factors based on the Singapore Ministry of Health Clinical Practice Guidelines for Diabetes Mellitus 1/2014 have to undergo OGTT
[c]$P < 0.001$ compared to universal screening

(95% CI 1.32–2.03) increases in risk for birth weight, neonatal percentage body fat, and sum of skinfolds greater than the 90th centile, respectively [21]. Each unit increase in gestational fasting glucose in non-obese mothers was further associated with higher weight [β = 0.08 (95% CI 0.008–0.16)] and BMI of the child [β = 0.08 (95% CI 0.003–0.15)], as well as a 36% higher risk of being overweight in the first 3 years of life (95% CI 1.10–1.68) [22]. Equally troubling is that infants of mothers with GDM tended to have greater abdominal adipose tissue in all three depots (internal, superficial, and deep subcutaneous), as observed through MRI scans at 1 week of life, suggesting that GDM influences metabolically important adipose depots at birth, even in the absence of overt neonatal macrosomia. The relationship between maternal gestational glycemia and offspring body composition [23] might be linked to the increasing prevalence of obesity and metabolic disease in adulthood. GUSTO continues to monitor the implications of these findings. Maternal glucose tolerance at mid-gestation predicted a reduced degree of coordinated neural activity in the electrophysiology neurocognitive assessment of their infants during an attentional task at both 6 and 18 months of age. The electrophysiologically measured evoked potential maximum amplitude difference (oddball-standard) was lower in the left hemisphere of offspring born to GDM mothers at both 6 [adjusted difference GDM vs. control: −0.62 vs. +0.15 μV, $P = 0.039$] and 18 months of age [adjusted difference GDM vs. control: −0.66 vs. +0.27 μV, $P = 0.039$]. Two-hour maternal glucose levels were associated with the difference in the evoked potential maximum amplitude at both 6 [adjusted β = −0.19 (95% CI −0.42 to 0.04) μV] and 18 months [adjusted β = −0.27 (95% CI −0.49 to −0.06) μV]. These findings suggest that antenatal maternal glycemia levels directly influence offspring neural activity in a test that predicts vulnerability for attentional difficulties such as attention deficit hyperactivity disorder (ADHD) [24]. This too argues for greater attention to glycemic control during pregnancy.

Following delivery, the subsequent development of type 2 diabetes mellitus occurs within 5 years in around 11% of women who had gestational diabetes, the majority of whom are not diagnosed or followed up under the current system. A meta-analysis performed on 20 selected studies worldwide showed that women who had GDM were sevenfold more likely to develop T2DM later in life when compared to those without such medical history [relative risk 7.43 (95% CI 4.79–11.51)] [25]. In GUSTO, preliminary analyses showed that women who were diagnosed with GDM during pregnancy had over 11 times the risk of developing type 2 diabetes (11.0%) compared to those who were not diagnosed with GDM (0.7%) within 5 years of the index pregnancy, after adjusting for ethnicity, mother's age at delivery, parity at delivery, prepregnancy BMI, family history of diabetes, and personal history of hypertension at delivery *(unpublished observation)*. Universal screening of women for GDM and lifelong post-diagnosis follow-up and surveillance of women with GDM and their offspring can provide an early window of opportunity to improve the long-term health and human capacity of Singaporeans. Current clinical practice should be reviewed to ensure appropriate diagnosis and follow-up of GDM and is a primary preventive strategy that could help tackle the epidemic of NCDs in Singapore, both for women and their children. We submitted a formal report to the Ministry of Health in September 2015, which has already influenced the GDM screening policy in the three public maternity units in Singapore, resulting in universal screening for GDM in all pregnant women regardless of known risk factors. This practice is formally adopted by the Ministry of Health in February 2017. We will continue to review the GDM diagnostic criteria that are suitable for the local population and work with the Ministry to set up a national GDM registry for long-term follow-up and surveillance.

8.3.2 Maternal Emotional Well-Being

Prior research, as well as our findings in GUSTO, strongly suggests that depression and anxiety in women during pregnancy have important effects on birth outcomes and fetal brain development [26–28]. GUSTO mothers were assessed with the Spielberger State-Trait Anxiety Inventory (STAI) and Edinburgh Postnatal Depression Scale (EPDS) at 26–28 weeks of gestation. Within the first 2 weeks of birth, a subset of the GUSTO neonates underwent MRI, which was repeated at 6 months of age. This is the first study in the world to directly examine the impact of maternal mental health on fetal brain development. Our findings showed that there were very significant effects of maternal depression on the functional connectivity [29] and microstructure of the amygdala [30], as well as an influence of maternal anxiety on hippocampal growth [31] and cortico-limbic structures [32]. These effects cut across the normal population and included infants born to mothers with subclinical levels of emotional problems. The effects of maternal emotional state were evident in brain regions, and the connections between brain regions, which regulate cognitive and emotional function and which could then predict the subsequent risk for mental disorders and behavioral problems. In addition, the development of the prefrontal and parietal cortex, critical brain regions for executive functioning and sensory processing, of GUSTO neonates born to anxious mothers was modified by the catechol-*O*-methyltransferase (COMT) haplotype of the newborn [33]. An increased risk for anxiety may thus be transmitted from mother to fetus, where the effect may be dependent upon the infant's COMT genotype, indicating a gene-environment interaction. Furthermore, we found that maternal antenatal anxiety was correlated with negative infant temperamental traits at 3 months old [34].

Postpartum maternal mood also had significant effects on women's parenting behaviors and their children's early neurodevelopment [35, 36]. Interventions targeting maternal depression and anxiety may help to decrease the risk for psychiatric disorders in the offspring including anxiety, depressive disorders, and disruptive behaviors like impulsivity and attention deficit hyperactivity disorder. A formal report was submitted to the Ministry of Health in September 2015 to suggest that easy-to-administer screening tools be integrated into routine prenatal and postnatal care across all government and private maternity hospitals to identify women with high levels of depressive or anxiety symptoms embarking on pregnancies as well as in the stressful postnatal period. Women with significant symptoms or risk factors should be followed up with professional support by allied health personnel during pregnancy and continuity of care from hospital to home. Risk factors and social determinants for antenatal and postnatal anxiety and depression should be identified to provide targeted help for high-risk groups.

Coincidentally, and in line with our recommendations, the US Preventive Services Task Force (USPSTF) issued guidelines recommending screening adults, including pregnant and postpartum women, for depression in February 2016. A systematic approach to the implementation would allow proper diagnosis and management of the mother and their offspring [37].

Our continued work in this area has demonstrated the importance of maternal mental health and neurodevelopment, resulting in a funding award by the president for a social program on maternal mood. A nurturing environment during the child's early years is important. With further understanding of gene-environment interactions, our work could lead us further into the area of personalized disease prevention for mothers and children.

8.3.3 Antenatal Micronutrient Status

Seven observational studies included in a recent meta-analysis indicated that vitamin D deficiency (serum 25-hydroxyvitamin D (25OHD) <50 nmol/L) in pregnant women was associated with a higher incidence of GDM [OR 1.61 (95% CI 1.19–2.17)] [38]. In GUSTO, we found that 41.3% of the GUSTO women had 25OHD inadequacy ($\leq$75 nmol/L), and this was associated with higher fasting glucose [β = 0.08 mmol/L, (95% CI 0.01, 0.14)] at 26–28 weeks' gestation, especially in Malay women [β = 0.19 mmol/L (95% CI 0.04, 0.33)]. No significant relationship was observed between 2-h postprandial glucose concentrations and the incidence of GDM [39]. Other work from our EpiGen consortium collaborators in Southampton,

United Kingdom, has also shown that maternal vitamin D insufficiency was associated with lower body fat in the neonates but with greater body fat at 4 and 6 years of age [40], potentially acting through epigenetic changes [41].

Although other micronutrients, such as folate, had a low prevalence of deficiency among the pregnant women in the GUSTO study, women with probable antenatal depression had significantly lower plasma folate concentrations at 26–28 weeks' gestation than those without [42]. There was no significant association with probable postnatal depression. Conversely, higher plasma folate concentrations were associated with a longer duration of gestation at delivery [0.12 week per SD increase in folate (95% CI 0.02, 0.21)] and lower risk of preterm birth [OR 0.79 (95% CI 0.63, 1.00)].

Our findings, together with the work of the EpiGen consortium, have led to the Nutritional Intervention Preconception and during Pregnancy to maintain healthy glucosE levels and offspRing health (NiPPeR) clinical trial (ClinicalTrials.gov NCT02509988) (refer to Chap. 15), which will lead to important new knowledge for the development of better nutrition guidelines for prospective parents, pregnant women, infants, and children.

8.4 Future Plans

8.4.1 S-PRESTO

Questions arising from the GUSTO studies and elsewhere pointed toward the need to consider the preconceptual and early post-conceptual period. This led to the decision to establish the Singapore PREconception Study of long-Term maternal and child Outcomes (S-PRESTO) cohort. This longitudinal study aims to recruit 1000 women who wish to conceive and study an estimated 400 resulting pregnancies. Recruitment started in March 2015 and has been most encouraging in spite of a challenging biosample collection and phenotyping protocol. As of April 2018, we have completed recruitment of 1055 participants, of whom 440 have conceived and 235 of these women have delivered. The oldest S-PRESTO offspring is currently more than 2 years old. The study has the globally unique design of recruiting before pregnancy and undertaking extensive nutritional, metabolic, and neuroendophenotyping before pregnancy and in the first trimester. The core hypothesis of the study, in part based on GUSTO data, is that maternal metabolic state and endophenotype before and soon after conception have a major effect on offspring epigenotype and later phenotypic outcomes.

The value of the GUSTO, S-PRESTO, and NiPPeR deeply phenotyped and biosampled cohorts in academic terms is substantial as the preconception and early gestation periods of human development are poorly studied. Yet from the available clinical and comparative evidence, the preconception and early gestation periods may be the most critical time for optimal human development (Fig. 8.2).

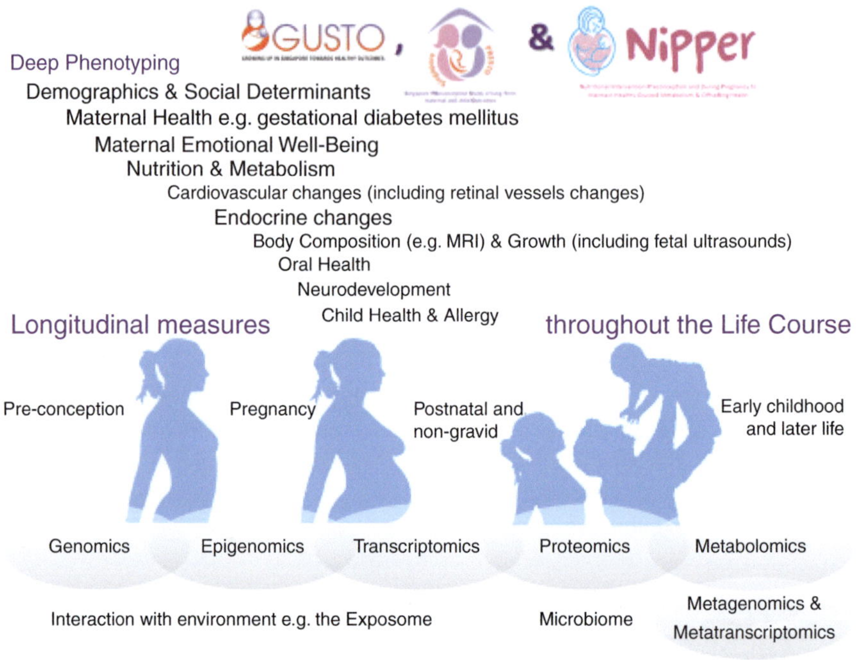

Fig. 8.2 Deep phenotyping and longitudinal measures in the GUSTO, S-PRESTO and NiPPeR studies

8.4.2 Birth Cohort Consortium of Asia (BiCCA)

The GUSTO team joined the Birth Cohort Consortium of Asia (BiCCA) in 2012 with the aim of creating an integrated platform to consolidate a comprehensive overview of birth cohorts in Asia to allow the exploration of differences in cohort findings between developed and developing Asian countries. As of December 2017, the consortium includes 27 birth cohorts in 13 Asian countries, including China, Taiwan, Japan, Korea, the Philippines, Vietnam, Malaysia, Singapore, Nepal, Mongolia, United Arab Emirates, Bangladesh, and Sri Lanka. BiCCA meetings occur on a yearly basis to discuss design, measurement, and analysis methods for various maternal and child health outcomes. BiCCA aims to combine and harmonize the data from its cohorts to give a larger sample size and improve the statistical power to evaluate associations between gene-environment interactions and assess important exposure-outcome relationship for rare health issues. In addition, through this enlarged set of data and extended diversity of participants, the international cooperation will provide a deeper insight into maternal and child health. The experiences shared and knowledge derived will help in identification of the priorities for health policymaking and organization of the next generation of birth cohorts.

8.5 Conclusion

GUSTO is distinctive in marrying neurodevelopmental, metabolic, and biological phenotyping with longitudinal biosampling. As the children in GUSTO enter school age, phenotyping now includes important linkages to the educational sector. It is one of the most detailed mother-offspring cohorts in Asia, and arguably no other cohort has the depth of phenotyping in infancy as these children have had. This has been supported by extensive genotyping, initial epigenotyping at birth, the collection of multiple biospecimens, and increasingly metabolomics and metagenomics. As the children enter puberty over the next 3 years, the potential for a range of definitive outcome measures in metabolic and cardiovascular state, body composition, cognition, and behaviors has emerged. The findings will be important in instituting preventive and intervention strategies targeting healthy childhood development, reducing the risk of metabolic and mental diseases, as well as enhancing human capacity.

Acknowledgments This research is supported by the Singapore National Research Foundation under its Translational and Clinical Research (TCR) Flagship Programme and administered by the Singapore Ministry of Health's National Medical Research Council (NMRC), Singapore-NMRC/TCR/004-NUS/2008; NMRC/TCR/012-NUHS/2014. Additional funding is provided by the Singapore Institute for Clinical Sciences, Agency for Science, Technology and Research (A*STAR), Singapore, and Nestec. Study sponsors were not involved in the design of the study, statistical analysis, and results interpretation. K. M. G. is supported by the National Institute for Health Research through the NIHR Southampton Biomedical Research Centre and by the European Union's Seventh Framework Programme (FP7/2007-2013) and projects EarlyNutrition and ODIN (Food-Based Solutions for Optimal Vitamin D Nutrition and Health through the Life Cycle) under grant agreements nos. 289346 and 613977.

The authors thank the GUSTO study group, which includes Allan Sheppard, Amutha Chinnadurai, Anne Eng Neo Goh, Anne Rifkin-Graboi, Anqi Qiu, Arijit Biswas, Bee Wah Lee, Birit F. P. Broekman, Boon Long Quah, Borys Shuter, Carolina Un Lam, Chai Kiat Chng, Cheryl Ngo, Choon Looi Bong, Christiani Jeyakumar Henry, Claudia Chi, Cornelia Yin Ing Chee, Yam Thiam Daniel Goh, Doris Fok, E. Shyong Tai, Elaine Tham, Elaine Quah Phaik Ling, Evelyn Xiu Ling Loo, Fabian Yap, Falk Mueller-Riemenschneider, George Seow Heong Yeo, Helen Chen, Heng Hao Tan, Hugo P. S. van Bever, Iliana Magiati, Inez Bik Yun Wong, Ivy Yee-Man Lau, Izzuddin Bin Mohd Aris, Jeevesh Kapur, Jenny L. Richmond, Jerry Kok Yen Chan, Joanna D. Holbrook, Joanne Yoong, Joao N. Ferreira., Jonathan Tze Liang Choo, Jonathan Y. Bernard, Joshua J. Gooley, Keith M. Godfrey, Kenneth Kwek, Kok Hian Tan, Krishnamoorthy Niduvaje, Kuan Jin Lee, Leher Singh, Lieng Hsi Ling, Lin Lin Su, Ling-Wei Chen, Lourdes Mary Daniel, Lynette Pei-Chi Shek, Marielle V. Fortier, Mark Hanson, Mary Foong-Fong Chong, Mary Rauff, Mei Chien Chua, Melvin Khee-Shing Leow, Michael Meaney, Mya Thway Tint, Neerja Karnani, Ngee Lek, Oon Hoe Teoh, P. C. Wong, Paulin Tay Straughan, Peter D. Gluckman, Pratibha Agarwal, Queenie Ling Jun Li, Rob M. van Dam, Salome A. Rebello, Seang-Mei Saw, See Ling Loy, S. Sendhil Velan, Seng Bin Ang, Shang Chee Chong, Sharon Ng, Shiao-Yng Chan, Shirong Cai, Shu-E Soh, Sok Bee Lim, Stella Tsotsi, Chin-Ying Stephen Hsu, Sue Anne Toh, Swee Chye Quek, Victor Samuel Rajadurai, Walter Stunkel, Wayne Cutfield, Wee Meng Han, Wei Wei Pang, Yap-Seng Chong, Yin Bun Cheung, Yiong Huak Chan, Yung Seng Lee, and Zhongwei Huang.

References

1. Horton R. Non-communicable diseases: 2015 to 2025. Lancet. 2013;381(9866):509–10.
2. World Health Organization. Global action plan for the prevention and control of noncommunicable diseases 2013-2020; 2013.
3. International Diabetes Federation. IDF diabetes atlas. 7th ed. Brussels: International Diabetes Federation; 2015.
4. Ministry of Health Singapore Epidemiology and Disease Control Department. Singapore: National Health Survey; 2010.
5. Teh AL, Pan H, Chen L, Ong ML, Dogra S, Wong J, et al. The effect of genotype and in utero environment on interindividual variation in neonate DNA methylomes. Genome Res. 2014;24(7):1064–74.
6. Gluckman PD, Hanson MA, Buklijas T. A conceptual framework for the developmental origins of health and disease. J Dev Orig Health Dis. 2010;1(1):6–18.
7. Misra A, Khurana L. Obesity-related non-communicable diseases: South Asians vs White Caucasians. Int J Obes (Lond). 2011;35(2):167–87.
8. Gujral UP, Pradeepa R, Weber MB, Narayan KM, Mohan V. Type 2 diabetes in South Asians: similarities and differences with white Caucasian and other populations. Ann N Y Acad Sci. 2013;1281:51–63.
9. Murgatroyd C, Spengler D. Epigenetics of early child development. Front Psych. 2011;2:16.
10. Paul AM. How the first nine months shape the rest of your life. Time 2010 Oct 4.
11. Soh SE, Tint MT, Gluckman PD, Godfrey KM, Rifkin-Graboi A, Chan YH, et al. Cohort profile: Growing Up in Singapore Towards Healthy Outcomes (GUSTO) birth cohort study. Int J Epidemiol. 2014;43(5):1401–9.
12. Feng Z. Stressed mums may have 'moody' babies. The Straits Times. 2015 Feb 16
13. Tang A. Babies exposed to two languages show better memory and learning ability: Study. The Straits Times. 2014 Sep 2.
14. Khalik S. Diabetes fight focuses on pregnant women. The Straits Times. 2016 Mar 29
15. Boh S. Pregnancy-time diabetes may be risky for babies. The Straits Times 2016 Nov 11.
16. Ministry of Education. MOE FY 2015 committee of supply debate—speech by Minister Heng Swee Keat. 2015 Mar 6.
17. Ministry of Education. Launch of the war on diabetes public engagement exercise—speech by Minister Ng Chee Meng. 2016 Sept 24.
18. Speech by Mr Teo Chee Hean, DPM, Coordinating Minister for National Security & Minister for Home Affairs, Chairman, NRF, Prime Minister's Office, Singapore at the Gala Dinner for the 30th Anniversary of IMCB. 2015 May 11.
19. Speech by Dr Lam Pin Min, Minister of State for Health, at the opening ceremony of the 10th Asia Pacific Congress in Maternal Fetal Medicine. 2014 Aug 22.
20. Chong YS, Cai S, Lin H, Soh SE, Lee YS, Leow MK, et al. Ethnic differences translate to inadequacy of high-risk screening for gestational diabetes mellitus in an Asian population: a cohort study. BMC Pregnancy Childbirth. 2014;14:345.
21. Aris IM, Soh SE, Tint MT, Liang S, Chinnadurai A, Saw SM, et al. Effect of maternal glycemia on neonatal adiposity in a multiethnic Asian birth cohort. J Clin Endocrinol Metab. 2014;99(1):240–7.
22. Aris IM, Soh SE, Tint MT, Saw SM, Rajadurai VS, Godfrey KM, et al. Associations of gestational glycemia and prepregnancy adiposity with offspring growth and adiposity in an Asian population. Am J Clin Nutr. 2015;102(5):1104–12.
23. Logan KM, Gale C, Hyde MJ, Santhakumaran S, Modi N. Diabetes in pregnancy and infant adiposity: systematic review and meta-analysis. Arch Dis Child Fetal Neonatal Ed. 2017;102(1):F65–72.
24. Cai S, Qiu A, Broekman BF, Wong EQ, Gluckman PD, Godfrey KM, et al. The influence of gestational diabetes on neurodevelopment of children in the first two years of life: a prospective study. PLoS One. 2016;11(9):e0162113.

25. Bellamy L, Casas JP, Hingorani AD, Williams D. Type 2 diabetes mellitus after gestational diabetes: a systematic review and meta-analysis. Lancet. 2009;373(9677):1773–9.
26. Alder J, Fink N, Bitzer J, Hosli I, Holzgreve W. Depression and anxiety during pregnancy: a risk factor for obstetric, fetal and neonatal outcome? A critical review of the literature. J Matern Fetal Neonatal Med. 2007;20(3):189–209.
27. Grote NK, Bridge JA, Gavin AR, Melville JL, Iyengar S, Katon WJ. A meta-analysis of depression during pregnancy and the risk of preterm birth, low birth weight, and intrauterine growth restriction. Arch Gen Psychiatry. 2010;67(10):1012–24.
28. Barker ED, Jaffee SR, Uher R, Maughan B. The contribution of prenatal and postnatal maternal anxiety and depression to child maladjustment. Depress Anxiety. 2011;28(8):696–702.
29. Qiu A, Anh TT, Li Y, Chen H, Rifkin-Graboi A, Broekman BF, et al. Prenatal maternal depression alters amygdala functional connectivity in 6-month-old infants. Transl Psychiatry. 2015;5:e508.
30. Rifkin-Graboi A, Bai J, Chen H, Hameed WB, Sim LW, Tint MT, et al. Prenatal maternal depression associates with microstructure of right amygdala in neonates at birth. Biol Psychiatry. 2013;74(11):837–44.
31. Qiu A, Rifkin-Graboi A, Chen H, Chong YS, Kwek K, Gluckman PD, et al. Maternal anxiety and infants' hippocampal development: timing matters. Transl Psychiatry. 2013;3:e306.
32. Rifkin-Graboi A, Meaney MJ, Chen H, Bai J, Hameed WB, Tint MT, et al. Antenatal maternal anxiety predicts variations in neural structures implicated in anxiety disorders in newborns. J Am Acad Child Adolesc Psychiatry. 2015;54(4):313–21 e2.
33. Qiu A, Tuan TA, Ong ML, Li Y, Chen H, Rifkin-Graboi A, et al. COMT haplotypes modulate associations of antenatal maternal anxiety and neonatal cortical morphology. Am J Psychiatry. 2015;172(2):163–72.
34. Chong SC, Broekman BF, Qiu A, Aris IM, Chan YH, Rifkin-Graboi A, et al. Anxiety and depression during pregnancy and temperament in early infancy: findings from a multi-ethnic, Asian, prospective birth cohort study. Infant Ment Health J. 2016;37(5):584–98.
35. Logsdon MC, Wisner KL, Pinto-Foltz MD. The impact of postpartum depression on mothering. J Obstet Gynecol Neonatal Nurs. 2006;35(5):652–8.
36. Koutra K, Chatzi L, Bagkeris M, Vassilaki M, Bitsios P, Kogevinas M. Antenatal and postnatal maternal mental health as determinants of infant neurodevelopment at 18 months of age in a mother-child cohort (Rhea Study) in Crete. Greece Soc Psychiatry Psychiatr Epidemiol. 2013;48(8):1335–45.
37. Siu AL, Force USPST, Bibbins-Domingo K, Grossman DC, Baumann LC, Davidson KW, et al. Screening for depression in adults: US Preventive Services Task Force Recommendation Statement. JAMA. 2016;315(4):380–7.
38. Poel YH, Hummel P, Lips P, Stam F, van der Ploeg T, Simsek S. Vitamin D and gestational diabetes: a systematic review and meta-analysis. Eur J Intern Med. 2012;23(5):465–9.
39. Loy SL, Lek N, Yap F, Soh SE, Padmapriya N, Tan KH, et al. Association of maternal vitamin D status with glucose tolerance and caesarean section in a multi-ethnic Asian cohort: the Growing Up in Singapore Towards Healthy Outcomes Study. PLoS One. 2015;10(11):e0142239.
40. Crozier SR, Harvey NC, Inskip HM, Godfrey KM, Cooper C, Robinson SM, et al. Maternal vitamin D status in pregnancy is associated with adiposity in the offspring: findings from the Southampton Women's Survey. Am J Clin Nutr. 2012;96(1):57–63.
41. Godfrey KM, Sheppard A, Gluckman PD, Lillycrop KA, Burdge GC, McLean C, et al. Epigenetic gene promoter methylation at birth is associated with child's later adiposity. Diabetes. 2011;60(5):1528–34.
42. Chong MF, Wong JX, Colega M, Chen LW, van Dam RM, Tan CS, et al. Relationships of maternal folate and vitamin B12 status during pregnancy with perinatal depression: the GUSTO study. J Psychiatr Res. 2014;55:110–6.

Chapter 9
The Hokkaido Study on Environment and Children's Health

Reiko Kishi, Atsuko Araki, Chihiro Miyashita, Sumitaka Kobayashi, Ryu Miura, and Machiko Minatoya

Abstract The Hokkaido Study on Environment and Children's Health is an ongoing study of two birth cohorts: the Sapporo cohort and the Hokkaido cohort. Our primary goals are (1) to examine the possible effects of low-level environmental chemical exposures, (2) to follow childhood development through a longitudinal observation study, (3) to identify a high-risk group classified by genetic susceptibility, and (4) to identify any additive effects. Maternal and cord blood were collected for an environmental chemical exposure assessment of dioxins, polychlorinated biphenyls, organochlorine pesticides, perfluoroalkyl substances, phthalates, bisphenol A, and methylmercury. Assessments of health outcomes regarding birth size, neurodevelopment, asthma, allergies and infectious diseases, and hormone levels were conducted, along with observation of the children's growth. Both genetic and epigenetic analyses were also conducted to examine the effects of environmental chemical exposures on a genetically susceptible population and on DNA methylation. Our study suggests that prenatal environmental chemical exposure affects birth size, hormone balance, neurodevelopment, and immune function, even at relatively low levels. Furthermore, specific genotypes may modify the effects of chemical exposure on health outcomes. Epigenetics, such as DNA methylation, may explain in part the mechanism of action.

Keywords Birth cohort · Health effects · Children · Early life exposure · Environmental chemicals · Genetic susceptibility · Epigenetics

---

R. Kishi (✉) · A. Araki · C. Miyashita · S. Kobayashi · R. Miura · M. Minatoya
Hokkaido University Center for Environmental and Health Sciences, WHO Collaborating Centre for Environmental Health and Prevention of Chemical Hazards, Sapporo, Japan
e-mail: rkishi@med.hokudai.ac.jp

F. Sata et al. (eds.), *Pre-emptive Medicine: Public Health Aspects of Developmental Origins of Health and Disease*, Current Topics in Environmental Health and Preventive Medicine, https://doi.org/10.1007/978-981-13-2194-8_9

Abbreviations

ADHD-RS	Attention deficit hyperactivity disorder-rating scale
AHR	Aromatic hydrocarbon receptor
ASQ	Autism screening questionnaire
ATS-DLD	American Thoracic Society-Division of Lung Disease classifications
BiCCA	Birth Cohort Consortium of Asia
BMI	Body mass index
BPA	Bisphenol A
BSID-II	The Bayley Scales of Infant Development-Second Edition
CBCL	Child behavior checklist
CI	Confidence interval
Conners 3P	Conner's third Edition for Parents
CYP	Cytochrome P450
DCDQ	Developmental Coordination Disorder Questionnaire
DDST	The Denver Developmental Screening Test
DEHP	Di(2-ethylhexyl) phthalate
DHEA	Dehydroepiandrostenedione
DL-PCBs	Dioxin-like polychlorinated biphenyls
DOHaD	Developmental Origins of Health and Disease
EES	The Evaluation of Environmental Stimulation
FT4	Free thyroxine
FTII	The Fagan Test of Infant Intelligence
GC/MS	Gas chromatography/mass spectrometry
GSTM1	Glutathione S-transferase mu 1
IGF2	Insulin-like growth factor 2
ISAAC	International Study of Asthma and Allergies in Childhood
J-PSAI	Japanese Pre-school Activities Inventory
K-ABC	The Kaufman Assessment Battery for Children
KIDS	Kinder Infant Development Scale
KWCST	Wisconsin Card Sorting Test (Keio version)
LBW	Low birth weight
LC-MS/MS	Liquid chromatography-tandem mass spectrometry
LINE1	Long interspersed element 1
M-CHAT	Modified Checklist for Autism Toddlers
MDI	Mental Development Index
Me-Hg	Methylmercury
MEHP	Mono(2-ethylhexyl) phthalate
MTHFR	5,10-methylenetetrahydrofolate reductase
NQO1	Reduced nicotinamide adenine dinucleotide phosphate (NADPH):quinone oxidase 1
PCDD/PCDF	Polychlorinated dibenzo-p-dioxin/polychlorinated dibenzofuran
PFASs	Perfluoroalkyl substances
PFOA	Perfluorooctanoate

PFOS	Perfluorooctanesulfonic acid
PI	Ponderal index
PRL	Prolactin
SCQ	Social Communication Questionnaire
SDQ	Strengths and Difficulties Questionnaire
SES	Social economic status
SGA	Small for gestational age
SNPs	Single nucleotide polymorphisms
T/E2	Testosterone/estradiol ratio
TEQ	Toxicity equivalency quantity
TSH	Thyroid-stimulating hormone
WAIS-R	The Wechsler Adult Intelligence Scale-Revised
WISC	The Wechsler Intelligence Scale for Children-Third Edition
XRCC1	X-ray cross-complementing gene 1

9.1 Introduction

In 1997, Colborn et al. warned of the dangers of environmental chemicals acting as endocrine disruptors, eventually leading to impairments in reproductive capacity [1]. Since that warning, a myriad of animal and epidemiological studies have been conducted to evaluate the adverse health effects of these endocrine-disrupting chemicals [2–4]. Currently, these chemicals are considered to contribute to numerous adverse health effects, including growth retardation of fetuses and infants, disturbances in neurodevelopment, alteration in thyroid and reproductive hormones, and disruption of immune and reproductive systems. Additionally, these chemicals may exert genetic or epigenetic effects when metabolized. In 1986, Barker and Osmond observed a relationship between poor nutrition in early life and a later risk of ischemic heart disease [5]. This observation had linked the importance of the intrauterine and early childhood nutritional environment, with the risk of disease in later life. Today, these criteria have been expanded from birth weight to encompass fetal and infantile development entirely which, in turn, has led to the establishment of the Developmental Origins of Health and Disease (DOHaD) hypothesis [6, 7].

Several birth cohort studies have been established in many different countries in recent years; however, few reports have been published on the relationship between low-level environmental exposures and adverse birth outcomes. In the field of infant development, variations in the human genome and their modifications on the effect of hazardous environment exposures (gene-environment integration) have not been thoroughly investigated. Therefore, the Hokkaido Study on Environment and Children's Health was established to investigate the effects of environmental exposure, combined with genetic predisposition, on development and health during the prenatal period, infancy, and early childhood. The study was primarily concerned with (1) examining the possible negative effects of perinatal environmental chemical exposures on birth outcomes; (2) following the development of allergies, infectious diseases, and neuro-

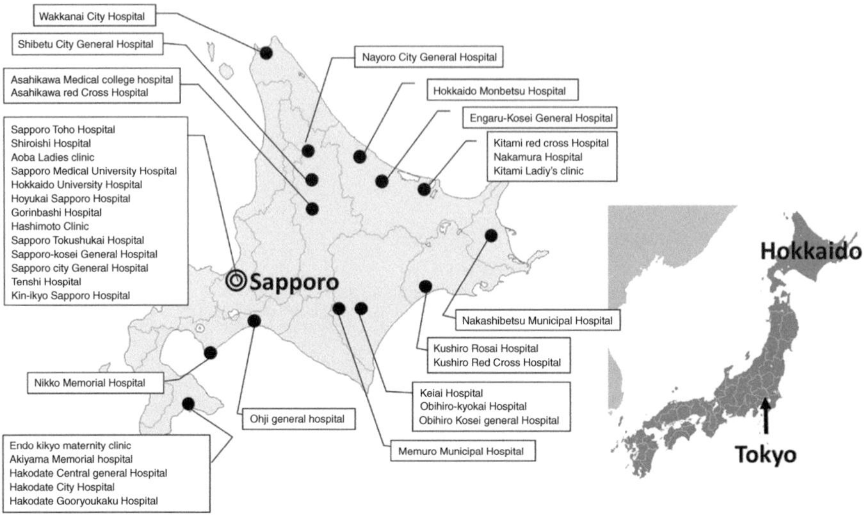

Fig. 9.1 The geographical distributions of the collaborating hospitals and clinics in Hokkaido, Japan

developmental disorders; (3) identifying high-risk groups with genetic susceptibilities to environmental chemicals; and (4) investigating the trans-generational epigenetic effects of environmental chemicals. Our final goal was to provide scientific evidence for health policies, based on human epidemiological data.

9.1.1 Study Areas and Participants

The Hokkaido study consists of two birth cohorts: the Sapporo cohort and the Hokkaido cohort [8–10]. In the Sapporo cohort, 514 pregnant women aged between 23 and 35 weeks of gestation, and planning to give birth at the Toho Hospital in Sapporo City between July 2002 and October 2005, were enrolled. In the Hokkaido (large-scale) cohort, pregnant women before 13 weeks of gestational age who had visited one of the associated hospitals or clinics in the Hokkaido prefecture (shown in Fig. 9.1) were enrolled for the period from February 2003 to March 2012. The fixed dataset at the end of 2015 included 20,926 women. Both the Sapporo cohort and the Hokkaido cohort studies were conducted with written informed consent of all participants. The institutional ethical board for human gene and genome studies at Hokkaido University Center for Environmental and Health Sciences and Hokkaido University Graduate School of Medicine approved the study protocol.

9.1.2 Follow-Up and Outcome Measures

The follow-up design for the study, including updated information, is described in Table 9.1.

Table 9.1 Design of the Hokkaido study

	Prenatal		Postnatal										
The Sapporo cohort		Third trimester	At birth	1 month	6–7 months	18 months		3.5 years			7 years		12 years
Specimens/ samples		Maternal blood	Cord blood	Breast milk									Child urine
			Maternal hair										
Health data		Baseline question-naire	Birth record		Develop-mental examination (BSID-II, FTII, EES)	Develop-mental examination (BSID-II, DDST, EES)		Developmental examination (K-ABC, WAIS-R, EES, CBCL)			Develop-mental examination (WISC-III, WCST-KFS, CBCL, J-PSAI)		Puberty onset
					Medical history	Medical history		Medical history			Medical history		
						ISAAC		ISAAC			ISAAC		
												2D/4D	
The Hokkaido cohort	First trimester	Third trimester	At birth	4 months	1 year	1.5 years	2 years	3 years	4 years	5–6 years	7 years	8 years	12 years
Specimens/ samples	Maternal blood	Maternal blood	Maternal blood								Child urine		Child urine

(continued)

Table 9.1 (continued)

	Prenatal		Postnatal										
			Cord blood								House dust		
Health data	Baseline question-naire		Birth record		Medical history		Medical history		Medical history	Medical history	Medical history		
					Physical growth	Physical growth		Physical growth		Physical growth	Physical growth	Physical growth	Physical growth
Allergies						ISAAC, ATS-DLD		ISAAC		ISAAC		ISAAC	
Neurodeve-lopment							M-CHAT		KIDS		SDQ, DCDQ, SCQ, ADHD-RS		ASQ
Life event, ADHD-RS, Conners3P, CBCL, WISC-IV													
Family factors				Parental smoking	Parental smoking	SES	Parental smoking	SES	Parental smoking	Parental smoking	Parental smoking	EES	
											2D/4D	J-PSAI	Puberty onset

ADHD-RS attention deficit hyperactivity disorder-rating scale, *ASQ* autism screening questionnaire, *ATS-DLD* American Thoracic Society-Division of Lung Disease classification, *BSID-II* the Bayley Scales of Infant Development-Second Edition, *CBCL* child behavior checklist, *Conners 3P* Conner's third Edition for Parents, *DCDQ* Developmental Coordination Disorder Questionnaire, *SCQ* Social Communication Questionnaire, *DDST* the Denver Developmental Screening Tests, *FTII* the Fagan Test of Infant Intelligence, *EES* the Evaluation of Environmental Stimulation, *ISAAC* the International Study of Asthma and Allergies in Childhood, *J-PSAI* Japanese Pre-school Activities Inventory, *K-ABC* the Kaufman Assessment Battery for Children, *KIDS* Kinder Infant Development Scale, *KWCST* Wisconsin Card Sorting Test (Keio version), *SDQ* Strengths and Difficulties Questionnaire, *SES* social economic status, *M-CHAT* Modified Checklist for Autism Toddlers, *WAIS-R* the Wechsler Adult Intelligence Scale-Revised, *WISC* the Wechsler Intelligence Scale for Children-Third Edition

In the Sapporo cohort study, we focused on child growth, neurodevelopment, allergy, and infectious diseases. A self-administered questionnaire was completed at the time of enrolment to obtain maternal and paternal baseline information. Maternal and infant birth records were obtained from the hospital at the time of birth. Follow-up questionnaires were administered at 6 months, 18 months, 3.5 years, and 7 years of age, which included relevant information regarding the medical history of asthma, allergies, and infectious diseases. At 7 years of age, the International Study of Asthma and Allergies in Childhood (ISAAC) criteria was used to determine if the children had allergies [11]. At 12 years of age, information on timing of puberty was collected. Neurodevelopmental examinations of the children were performed at 6–7 months, 18 months, 3.5 years, and 7 years of age. Used test batteries and questionnaires for the neurodevelopment are mentioned in Table 9.1.

In the Hokkaido cohort study, we focused on assessing the prevalence of birth defects, asthma and allergies, and neurodevelopmental disorders. Medical records of the parents and children were obtained from the physicians at the participating hospitals or clinics, including information about gestational age, birth weight, and any birth defects at delivery or at the end of pregnancy. In addition to basic information such as child height and weight, regular health checkup data, dietary habits, and parental smoking history, further information was collected regarding allergies and infections at 1, 2, 4, and 7 years of age. Information regarding allergies was obtained using the ISAAC and the American Thoracic Society-Division of Lung Disease (ATS-DLD) classifications [12]. At 8 years of age, information regarding any neurodevelopmental disorders, including attention deficit hyperactivity disorder, was collected. Later, the investigation was expanded to include social economic status (SES) and childhood behavioral problems at the subpopulation level of the Hokkaido cohort at 1.5 years, at 3 years, and at 5–6 years of age, as shown in Table 9.1. At 12 years of age, information regarding timing of puberty was collected.

9.1.3 Specimen Collection, Exposure, and Biochemical Measurements

In the Sapporo cohort study, maternal blood samples were collected at the time of the hospital examination following recruitment, between the 23rd and the 35th week of gestation. Cord blood and the placenta samples were taken immediately after delivery. Maternal hair samples and breast milk were also collected after delivery. The levels of 29 congeners of dioxins and dioxin-like polychlorinated biphenyls (DL-PCBs), 58 congeners of the other PCBs, and 5 congeners of hydroxylated PCBs in maternal blood and breast milk were measured using high-resolution gas chromatography (GC)/high-resolution mass spectrometry (MS) [13–15]. The toxicity equivalency quantity (TEQ) levels were calculated by multiplying the levels of individual congeners by their toxic equivalency factor values, as derived from WHO 2005 guidelines [16]. Perfluorooctanesulfonic acid (PFOS) and perfluorooctanoate (PFOA) levels in both maternal blood and in cord blood were analyzed using liquid chromatography-tandem mass spectrometry (LC-MS/MS) [17]. The levels of persistent organochlorine pesticides in maternal blood were analyzed using gas chromatography-negative ion chemical ionization mass spectrometry and GC/HRMS [18]. To determine maternal phthalate ester exposure, mono(2-ethylhexyl) phthalate (MEHP) (a primary metabolite of di(2-ethylhexyl) phthalate [DEHP]) levels in maternal blood were analyzed using GC/MS [19, 20]. Bisphenol A (BPA) concentrations in maternal and cord blood were analyzed using isotope dilution LC-MS/MS [21]. Total mercury levels in maternal hair samples were measured [22]. Items measured as biochemical markers were thyroid-stimulating hormone (TSH) and free thyroxine (FT4) levels of the mother and newborn [23], nine fatty acids and triglyceride levels in the maternal plasma [20, 24], the levels of cord serum IgE and IgA [25], the total and high molecular weight adiponectin and leptin [26, 27], and seven key steroid and five reproductive hormones [19, 28, 29].

In the Hokkaido cohort study, maternal blood samples were collected during the first and the third trimester and at delivery. Cord blood samples were taken immediately after delivery. Simultaneous analysis of 11 perfluoroalkyl substances (PFASs) in maternal plasma was perfumed with ultra-performance high performance LC-MS/MS at the Research Faculty of Agriculture, Hokkaido University [30]. Based on self-reports and plasma cotinine levels, and using the receiver operating characteristic curve, a cutoff value of 11.48 and 0.21 ng/mL was established for separating smokers and exposed non-smokers, respectively, from unexposed non-smokers. Maternal serum was also used to measure folic acid levels [31, 32].

9.1.4 Genetic Analysis

Single nucleotide polymorphisms (SNPs) were determined for both mothers and children in the Sapporo and the Hokkaido cohorts. Determination of SNPs was carried out using TaqMan PCR methods and the nanofluidic integrated fluidic circuit-based genotyping system for medium-throughput multiplexing, known as dynamic array (Fluidigm Corporation, South San Francisco, CA, USA) [33–36]. In the Sapporo cohort, DNA methylation in the genes of insulin-like growth factor 2 (IGF2), H19, and long interspersed element 1 (LINE1) DNA was measured from the cord blood samples of the offspring using pyrosequencing by the PyroMark Q24 system (Qiagen), and data were analyzed using the Pyro Q-CpG software (Qiagen) [37]. Cord blood DNA methylation at more than 450,000 CpGs was quantified, using Infinium HumanMethylation 450 BeadChip (Illumina, San Diego, CA, USA), according to the manufacturer's protocol [38, 39].

9.2 Findings from the Hokkaido Study

9.2.1 Effect of Prenatal Environmental Chemical Exposures on Birth Outcomes

9.2.1.1 Study Population and Birth Outcomes

In the Sapporo cohort, the prevalence of preterm, low birth weight (LBW), and small for gestational age (SGA) [40] was 5.6%, 5.8%, and 6.2%, respectively, among 497 singleton pregnancies. In the Hokkaido cohort, follow-up rate was 94.1%. After excluding 121 participants, who requested not to have their data used, the data of 20,805 participants was used in the analyses. The incidence of spontaneous abortion, stillbirths, and preterm births was 1.1%, 0.3%, and 4.9%, respectively. We observed LBW and macrosomia in 9.0% and 1.0% of births, respectively. The prevalence of SGA and term SGA was 7.0% and 6.5%, respectively.

9.2.1.2 Chemical Exposure Levels

Median levels of total TEQ and total PCBs in maternal blood were 13.9 pg/g lipid and 107 ng/g lipid, respectively. Median *p,p*'-dichlorodiphenyldichloroethylene level was 651.99 ng/g wet. The median PFOS and PFOA levels were 5.20 and 1.30 ng/mL, respectively. The median concentration of MEHP was 9.95 ng/mL. The concentration (detection percentages above detection limit) of BPA in maternal and cord blood was 0.057 ng/mL (68.8%) and 0.051 ng/mL (76.3%), respectively. The methylmercury (Me-Hg) concentration in maternal hair was 1.40 μg/g. In the Hokkaido cohort, the concentration of 11 PFASs in the third trimester maternal plasma was measured. The exposure levels were relatively low in the Hokkaido study when compared to the other countries.

9.2.1.3 Birth Size

The effects of exposure to polychlorinated dibenzo-p-dioxin/polychlorinated dibenzofuran (PCDD/PCDF) and dioxin-like PCB, PFOS, and PFOA on birth size are noted in the 2012 cohort profile [8]. Associations of PCBs and Me-Hg exposures with birth size were analyzed using multiple regression analysis, with adjustment for confounding factors. There was no overall association of any of MEHP, PCBs, or Me-Hg concentrations, with birth weight, birth length, chest circumference, or head circumference [27, 41]. Maternal PFOS and PFOA levels and cord blood adipokine levels were investigated. Only PFOS, but not PFOA, was positively associated with cord blood total adiponectin levels. PFOS and adiponectin levels showed marginal dose-response relationship [26]. Associations of prenatal MEHP with cord blood adipokine levels were also investigated. The MEHP level was positively associated with the adiponectin level among boys and was negatively associated with the leptin level among girls. The MEHP level was negatively associated with the ponderal index only in girls, which could be due to decreased leptin level. The results suggested that prenatal DEHP exposure may be associated with cord blood adipokine and with birth size [27].

9.2.2 The Effects on Hormone Levels at Birth, Alongside Neurodevelopmental Disorders, Allergies, and Infectious Diseases

9.2.2.1 Thyroid Hormones

Maternal PFOS levels were inversely correlated with maternal serum TSH levels and positively associated with infant serum TSH levels, whereas maternal PFOA levels showed no significant relationship with TSH or FT4 levels of mothers and infants [23]. On the other hand, for MEHP and BPA levels, we did not find any associations between prenatal exposures and infant thyroid hormone levels [42, 43].

9.2.2.2 Steroid and Reproductive Hormones

Reproductive and steroid hormones are essential for not only sex differentiation and maturation but also for regulating homeostasis in metabolism, growth, neurodevelopment, and the immune system [44–46]. Among boys, maternal PFOS levels were significantly associated with estradiol positively and the testosterone/estradiol ratio (T/E2), progesterone, and inhibin B levels inversely, whereas PFOA levels were positively associated with inhibin B levels. Among girls, there were significant inverse associations between PFOS levels and progesterone and prolactin (PRL) levels [29]. PFOS levels showed an inverse dose-response relationship with dehydroepiandrostenedione (DHEA) levels, whereas PFOA levels showed a positive association with DHEA levels [28]. Similar to PFOS, MEHP levels were associated with reduced levels of progesterone, inhibin B, and insulin-like factor 3, as well as a reduced T/E2 ratio, among boys [19]. MEHP levels were associated with reduced cortisol and cortisone levels, and glucocorticoid/adrenal androgen ratio, and increased DEHP levels, DHEA/androstenedione and cortisol/cortisone ratios [47]. The level of BPA in cord blood was inversely associated with PRL levels among boys, whereas it was positively associated among girls [43]. Our results indicate that prenatal exposure to PFOS, DEHP, and BPA may alter the steroid and reproductive hormones of children.

9.2.2.3 Neurodevelopment

Associations between prenatal PCDD/PCDF, PFAS, and DEHP exposures and child neurodevelopment were investigated [42, 48, 49]. At 6 months of age, after controlling for confounders, an inverse association between prenatal PCDD/PCDF levels with BSID-II scores was found among boys [49]. PFOA concentrations were inversely associated with the mental development index (MDI) scores of girls. The results suggest that the effects of exposure to PCDD/PCDF and PFOA differed between the sexes [48, 49]. No significant association between PFOS and MEHP concentrations and neurodevelopmental outcomes was observed in early infancy [42, 48].

The investigation was also expanded to cover other environmental factors, including SES, in association with childhood behavioral problems. A strengths and difficulties questionnaire [50, 51] was distributed between October 2014 and December 2015 to the subpopulation of the Hokkaido study aged 5 years at the time of the survey. The study found that prenatal socioeconomic factors were associated with a greater likelihood of developing childhood behavioral problems at preschool age in Japan [52].

9.2.2.4 Asthma, Allergies, and Infectious Diseases

The associations between PCBs and dioxin-like compounds, and the development of allergies and infectious diseases at 18 months of age, were assessed in the Sapporo cohort. After adjusting for confounders, relatively higher levels of PCDF were associated with a significantly increased risk of otitis media, especially among male infants [53].

In the Hokkaido cohort, the associations between prenatal exposure to PFASs, including long-chain compounds, and allergies at the ages of 12, 24, and 48 months were also investigated. At 12 months, after adjusting for confounding factors, no significant associations were observed between the prevalence of allergies and the levels of PFASs. At 24 and 48 months, an inverse dose-response relationship was obtained between prenatal exposure to PFASs and eczema, but no significant associations with wheezing were found [54, 55]. On the other hand, a dose-response relationship was obtained between PFAS levels and total infectious diseases [56]. These results suggest that prenatal exposure to dioxins and PFAS may alter the immune functions of the infant.

9.2.3 High-Risk Group Classified by SNP Genetic Susceptibility

The association of maternal smoking during pregnancy and maternal genetic polymorphisms was examined in the Sapporo cohort and the Hokkaido cohort (Table 9.2) [31, 33, 57, 58]. In the Hokkaido cohort, when considered maternal genotypes

Table 9.2 Adverse effects of infant birth weight in relation to maternal environmental exposure and genetic polymorphisms being studied in the Hokkaido Study on Environment and Children's Health up to 2017

Environmental exposure	Maternal genetic polymorphism	Maternal risk genotypes	Reduction of birth weight	Ref.
Active smoking	*AHR* (G > A, Arg554Lys)	Arg/Arg	211 g ↓	[32]
Active smoking	*CYP1A1* (m1/m2)	m1/m2 + m2/m2	170 g ↓	
Active smoking	*GSTM1* (non-null/null)	Null	171 g ↓	
Active smoking	Combination with *AHR* (G > A, Arg554Lys) and *CYP1A1* (m1/m2)	Combination with Arg/Arg (*AHR*) and m1/m2 + m2/m2 (*CYP1A1*)	315 g ↓	
Active smoking	Combination with *CYP1A1* (m1/m2) and *GSTM1* (non-null/null)	Combination with m1/m2 + m2/m2 (*CYP1A1*) and null (*GSTM1*)	237 g ↓	
Active smoking	*NQO1* (C > T, Pro187Ser)	Pro/Pro	159 g ↓	[57]
Active smoking	*CYP2E1* (c1/c2)	c1/c1	195 g ↓	
Active smoking	*MTHFR* (A1298C)	AA	105.69 g ↓	[30]
Active smoking	*CYP1A1* (A > G, Ile462Val)	AG/GG	62 g ↓	[56]
Active smoking	*XRCC1* (C > T, Arg194Trp)	CT/TT	59 g ↓	
Active smoking	Combination with *AHR*(G > A, Arg554Lys), *CYP1A1* (A > G, Ile462Val), and *XRCC1* (C > T, Arg194Trp)	Combination with GG (*AHR*) and AG/GG (*CYP1A1*) and CT/TT (*XRCC1*)	145 g ↓	
Dioxin (total TEQ)	*GSTM1* (non-null/null)	Null	345 g ↓	[59]

Ref., reference; ↓, reduction

Genes described in the table represents the genetic polymorphisms that are significantly associated with infant birth weight

Gene names: *AHR* aromatic hydrocarbon receptor, *CYP1A1* cytochrome P450 1A1, *GSTM1* glutathione S-transferase mu 1, *NQO1* reduced nicotinamide adenine dinucleotide phosphate (NADPH):quinone oxidase 1, *CYP2E1* cytochrome P450 2E1, *MTHFR* methylenetetrahydrofolate reductase, *XRCC1* X-ray cross-complementing gene 1

encoded with folate-metabolizing enzymes, among infants of pregnant women with the 5,10-methylenetetrahydrofolate reductase (*MTHFR*; A1298C)-AA genotype, infants born to women who smoked during the first trimester of pregnancy were 106.59 g smaller in birth weight than infants born to women who did not (Table 9.2) [31]. When using aforementioned definition of non-smokers and smokers using plasma cotinine levels, infants of smokers were 71 g smaller in birth weight than those of non-smokers. However, when we considered maternal genotypes encoding for PAH-metabolizing enzymes and DNA repair, we found that infants of smokers with combination of GG genotype of *AHR* Arg554Lys, AG/GG genotype of cytochrome P450 (*CYP*) *1A1* (Ile462Val), and CT/TT genotype of X-ray cross-complementing gene 1 (*XRCC1*; Arg194Trp) were 145 g smaller in birth weight than infants of non-smokers combined with *AHR*-GA/AA, *CYP1A1*-AA, and *XRCC1*-CC genotypes (Table 9.2) [57].

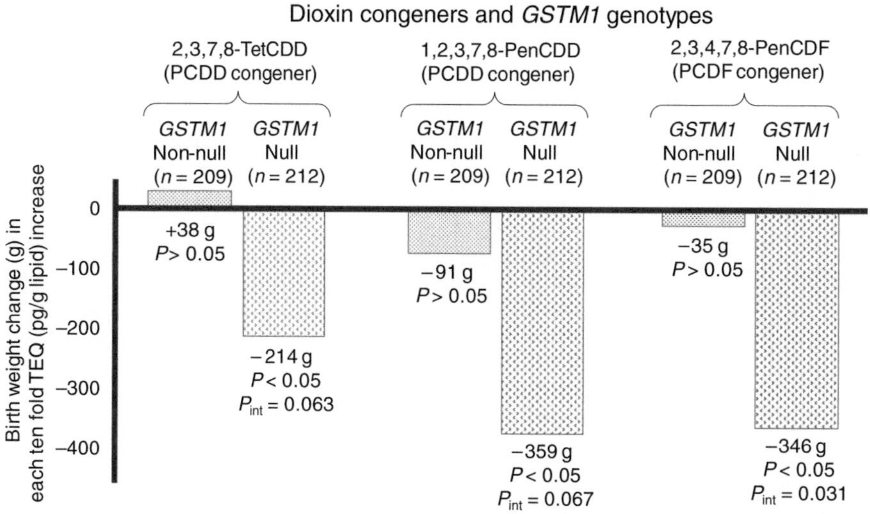

Fig. 9.2 Association of maternal PCDD and PCDF congeners and maternal GSTM1 (non-null/null) genotypes with reduction of infant birth weight in a multiple linear regression model ($N = 421$). The bar represents birth weight change (g) in increase for each tenfold increase in dioxin congener TEQ (pg/g lipid). Adjusted for maternal age, height, weight before pregnancy, caffeine intake, alcohol consumption during pregnancy, maternal smoking during pregnancy, parity, maternal education level, annual household income, in-shore fish intake during pregnancy, deep-sea fish intake during pregnancy, and blood sampling period. Interaction *P* value (P_{int}) was calculated using genotype, and each dioxin congener TEQ, for the two interaction variables between genotype and each congener TEQ. Original source of this figure is Kishi et al. (2017), and Kobayashi et al. (2017) [10, 60]

The association of maternal dioxin exposure during pregnancy and maternal genetic polymorphisms was examined in the Sapporo cohort. When considering dioxin-metabolizing enzymes/receptors, the adjusted mean TEQ levels of total of non-ortho PCB congeners and the total of mono-ortho PCB congeners in maternal blood were significantly different for genotypes of maternal AHR, as shown in Table 9.2 [59]. The adjusted mean TEQ levels of total of PCDD congeners and total of PCDF congeners in maternal blood were significantly different in certain genotypes of maternal *CYP1A1* [59]. Moreover, among 29 dioxin congeners, the reduction of infant birth weight for each tenfold increase of 2,3,7,8-tetrachlorinated dibenzo-p-dioxin, 1,2,3,7,8-pentachlorinated dibenzo-p-dioxin, and 2,3,4,7,8-pentachlorinated dibenzofuran TEQ in maternal blood during pregnancy was significantly different for maternal glutathione S-transferase mu 1 (*GSTM1*; non-null/null) genotypes (Fig. 9.2) [10, 60].

In this study, the maternal genetic polymorphisms in the *XRCC1* modified the association of maternal smoking with birth weight reduction [57]. Moreover, the results suggest that seven SNPs would be also the key genotypes of enzymes and receptors for the association of birth weight reduction [31, 32, 57, 58] but also with maternal dioxin exposure during pregnancy [60]. This study provides further genetic and environmental information about high-risk groups in the present and future generations that are susceptible to the risks in relation to environmental chemical exposures.

Table 9.3 Association between maternal PFAS concentrations and cord blood DNA methylation in multiple linear regression analyses ($N = 177$)

	IGF2 methylation (%)	*H19* methylation (%)	*LINE1* methylation (%)
	β (95% CI)	β (95% CI)	β (95% CI)
log (PFOS)	−0.56 (−1.56, 0.44)	−0.09 (−0.77, 0.59)	0.05 (−0.31, 0.42)
log (PFOA)	−0.73 (−1.44, −0.02)*	−0.08 (−0.57, 0.40)	−0.15 (−0.41, 0.10)

Abbreviations: β, partial regression coefficient, indicates methylation changes with log-unit increase in concentration; *CI*, confidence interval; *IGF2*, insulin growth factor 2; *LINE1*, long interspersed element 1; *PFAS*, perfluoroalkyl substances; *PFOA*, perfluorooctanoic acid; *PFOS*, perfluorooctane sulfonate

Adjusted for maternal age, maternal education, maternal smoking during pregnancy, infant sex, and maternal blood sampling period. *$P < 0.05$

9.2.4 Exploiting Epigenetic Effects on the Next Generation

We assessed the effect of prenatal PFAS exposure on cord blood IGF2, H19, and LINE1 methylation and evaluated whether association of PFAS exposure with birth size was mediated by DNA methylation [37]. Following further adjustment to multiple linear regression models, IGF2 methylation levels showed a significant negative association with log-unit increase in PFOA (partial regression coefficient = −0.73; 95% confidence interval [CI]: −1.44 to −0.02) but no significant effects on H19 or LINE1 methylation (Table 9.3). IGF2 methylation showed a significant association with the ponderal index at birth ($\beta = 0.17$; 95% CI: 0.06–0.27), but not with birth weight or birth length. We evaluated IGF2 methylation to test for any mediating effect (Fig. 9.3) [61] and concluded that reduced IGF2 methylation as a mediator could account for approximately 20% of the total effect (−0.55) of PFOA exposure on the ponderal index at birth (percent mediation = −0.11/−0.55 = 0.2) [62], which explained a 1.2% of variance in the ponderal index (R^2med = 0.012) [63]. It is remarkable that around one-fifth of the effects of prenatal PFOA exposure on the reduced ponderal index could be explained by methylation at only one gene, IGF2. IGF2 is essential for fetal growth, is expressed from the early embryonic stages, and continues to be expressed throughout fetal development. This result suggests that exposure to environmental chemicals in utero may affect infant health through their effects on DNA methylation.

9.3 Future Directions

First, investigating the effects of multiple chemical exposures is warranted. In their daily lives, humans are continuously exposed to multiple environmental chemicals. An estimation of the combined risks of these mixed effects is required. Secondly, this study suggests that exposure to environmental chemicals in utero may affect infant health through their effects on DNA methylation. A genome-wide study is currently being conducted to determine any long-term effects of prenatal exposure by way of epigenetic mechanisms. Thirdly, a long follow-up time of participants is

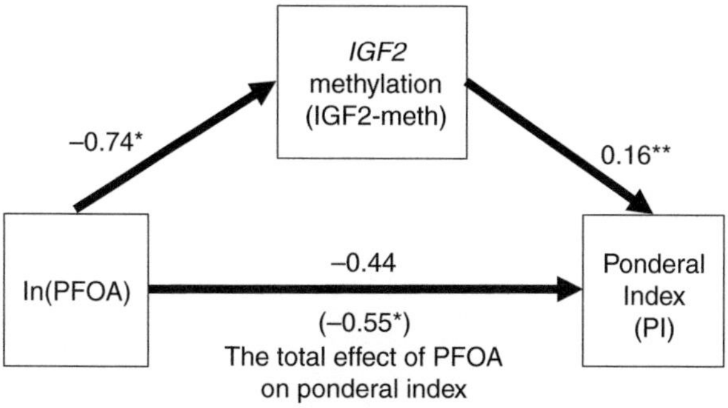

Fig. 9.3 Mediation analysis of the association between PFOA and IGF2 methylation and between PFOA and PI ($N = 175$). Regression coefficients of each path are described with arrows. The total effect of PFOA on PI is described within parentheses. A significant indirect effect of PFOA on PI through IGF2 hypomethylation was observed (indirect effect = −0.11; bias-corrected and accelerated confidence interval: −0.30 to −0.02). The IGF2 methylation as a mediator can account for approximately 20% of the total effect (percent mediation = 0.20). Maternal age, prepregnancy body mass index (BMI), parity, maternal education, maternal smoking during pregnancy, gestational age, infant sex, and maternal blood sampling period were adjusted (*$P < 0.05$ and **$P < 0.01$)

needed. The importance of the intrauterine and early childhood environment for understanding disease risk led to the establishment of the DOHaD hypothesis. Children in the Hokkaido study are now reaching the pubertal stage. The impact of fetal and early childhood exposures to environmental chemicals on neurobehavioral development, asthma and allergies, growth, and reproductive functions will be observed continuously and will require confirmation. Finally, the strengthening of the collaborations and integration with other birth cohort studies are important. The Birth Cohort Consortium of Asia (BiCCA) was launched in 2011, and, currently, 24 cohorts from 11 countries are participating (as of May, 2017) [64]. Although there are many challenges for facilitating different cohort studies, cooperative relationships will accelerate the establishment of new research among BiCCA members.

Acknowledgments We would like to express our appreciation to all the study participants and all the personnel in hospitals and clinics that collaborated with the Hokkaido study on environment and children's health. The Hokkaido study is supported by Grant-in-Aid for Scientific Research from the Japanese Ministry of Health, Labour and Welfare; Japan Society for the Promotion of Science; the Ministry of Education, Culture, Sports, Science and Technology; and Environment Research and Technology Development Fund.

References

1. Colborn T, Dumanoski D, Myers J. Our stolen future: are we threating our fertility, intelligence, and survival? A scientific detective story. New York: Plume; 1997.
2. Meeker JD. Exposure to environmental endocrine disruptors and child development. Arch Pediatr Adolesc Med. 2012;166(6):E1–7. https://doi.org/10.1001/archpediatrics.2012.241.

3. Schug TT, Janesick A, Blumberg B, et al. Endocrine disrupting chemicals and disease susceptibility. J Steroid Biochem Mol Biol. 2011;127(3–5):204–15. https://doi.org/10.1016/j.jsbmb.2011.08.007.
4. Wigle DT, Arbuckle TE, Turner MC, et al. Epidemiologic evidence of relationships between reproductive and child health outcomes and environmental chemical contaminants. J Toxicol Environ Health B Crit Rev. 2008;11(5–6):373–517. https://doi.org/10.1080/10937400801921320.
5. Barker DJ, Osmond C. Infant mortality, childhood nutrition, and ischaemic heart disease in England and Wales. Lancet. 1986;1(8489):1077–81.
6. Gluckman P, Hanson M. Early life origins of human health and disease. New York: Cambridge University Press; 2006.
7. Newman J, Ross M. Early life origins of human health and disease. Basel: Karger; 2009.
8. Kishi R, Kobayashi S, Ikeno T, et al. Ten years of progress in the Hokkaido birth cohort study on environment and children's health: cohort profile—updated 2013. Environ Health Prev Med. 2013;18(6):429–50. https://doi.org/10.1007/s12199-013-0357-3.
9. Kishi R, Sasaki S, Yoshioka E, et al. Cohort profile: the Hokkaido Study on Environment and Children's Health in Japan. Int J Epidemiol. 2011;40(3):611–8. https://doi.org/10.1093/ije/dyq071.
10. Kishi R, Araki A, Minatoya M, et al. The Hokkaido Birth Cohort Study on Environment and Children's Health: cohort profile—updated 2017. Environ Health Prev Med. 2017;22:46. https://doi.org/10.1186/s12199-017-0654-3.
11. Worldwide variation in prevalence of symptoms of asthma, allergic rhinoconjunctivitis, and atopic eczema: ISAAC. The International Study of Asthma and Allergies in Childhood (ISAAC) Steering Committee (1998). Lancet 351 (9111):1225–1232.
12. Nishima S, Chisaka H, Fujiwara T, et al. Surveys on the prevalence of pediatric bronchial asthma in Japan: a comparison between the 1982, 1992, and 2002 surveys conducted in the same region using the same methodology. Allergol Int. 2009;58(1):37–53. https://doi.org/10.2332/allergolint.O-08-550.
13. Todaka T, Hirakawa H, Kajiwara J, et al. Concentrations of polychlorinated dibenzo-p-dioxins, polychlorinated dibenzofurans, and dioxin-like polychlorinated biphenyls in blood collected from 195 pregnant women in Sapporo City, Japan. Chemosphere. 2007;69(8):1228–37. https://doi.org/10.1016/j.chemosphere.2007.05.083.
14. Todaka T, Hirakawa H, Kajiwara J, et al. Concentrations of polychlorinated dibenzo-p-dioxins, polychlorinated dibenzofurans, and dioxin-like polychlorinated biphenyls in blood and breast milk collected from 60 mothers in Sapporo City, Japan. Chemosphere. 2008;72(8):1152–8. https://doi.org/10.1016/j.chemosphere.2008.03.050.
15. Todaka T, Hori T, Hirakawa H, et al. Congener-specific analysis of non-dioxin-like polychlorinated biphenyls in blood collected from 195 pregnant women in Sapporo City, Japan. Chemosphere. 2008;73(6):923–31. https://doi.org/10.1016/j.chemosphere.2008.06.071.
16. Van den Berg M, Birnbaum LS, Denison M, et al. The 2005 World Health Organization reevaluation of human and Mammalian toxic equivalency factors for dioxins and dioxin-like compounds. Toxicol Sci. 2006;93(2):223–41. https://doi.org/10.1093/toxsci/kfl055.
17. Inoue K, Okada F, Ito R, et al. Perfluorooctane sulfonate (PFOS) and related perfluorinated compounds in human maternal and cord blood samples: assessment of PFOS exposure in a susceptible population during pregnancy. Environ Health Perspect. 2004;112(11):1204–7.
18. Kanazawa A, Miyasita C, Okada E, et al. Blood persistent organochlorine pesticides in pregnant women in relation to physical and environmental variables in The Hokkaido Study on Environment and Children's Health. Sci Total Environ. 2012;426:73–82. https://doi.org/10.1016/j.scitotenv.2012.02.073.
19. Araki A, Mitsui T, Miyashita C, et al. Association between maternal exposure to di(2-ethylhexyl) phthalate and reproductive hormone levels in fetal blood: the Hokkaido Study on Environment and Children's Health. PLoS One. 2014;9(10):e109039. https://doi.org/10.1371/journal.pone.0109039.

20. Jia X, Harada Y, Tagawa M, et al. Prenatal maternal blood triglyceride and fatty acid levels in relation to exposure to di(2-ethylhexyl)phthalate: a cross-sectional study. Environ Health Prev Med. 2015;20(3):168–78. https://doi.org/10.1007/s12199-014-0440-4.
21. Yamamoto J, Minatoya M, Sasaki S, et al. Quantifying bisphenol A in maternal and cord whole blood using isotope dilution liquid chromatography/tandem mass spectrometry and maternal characteristics associated with bisphenol A. Chemosphere. 2016;164:25–31. https://doi.org/10.1016/j.chemosphere.2016.08.001.
22. Miyashita C, Sasaki S, Saijo Y, et al. Demographic, behavioral, dietary, and socioeconomic characteristics related to persistent organic pollutants and mercury levels in pregnant women in Japan. Chemosphere. 2015;133:13–21. https://doi.org/10.1016/j.chemosphere.2015.02.062.
23. Kato S, Itoh S, Yuasa M, et al. Association of perfluorinated chemical exposure in utero with maternal and infant thyroid hormone levels in the Sapporo cohort of Hokkaido Study on the Environment and Children's Health. Environ Health Prev Med. 2016;21(5):334–44. https://doi.org/10.1007/s12199-016-0534-2.
24. Kishi R, Nakajima T, Goudarzi H, et al. The association of prenatal exposure to perfluorinated chemicals with maternal essential and long-chain polyunsaturated fatty acids during pregnancy and the birth weight of their offspring: the Hokkaido Study. Environ Health Perspect. 2015;123(10):1038–45. https://doi.org/10.1289/ehp.1408834.
25. Okada E, Sasaki S, Saijo Y, et al. Prenatal exposure to perfluorinated chemicals and relationship with allergies and infectious diseases in infants. Environ Res. 2012;112:118–25. https://doi.org/10.1016/j.envres.2011.10.003.
26. Minatoya M, Itoh S, Miyashita C, et al. Association of prenatal exposure to perfluoroalkyl substances with cord blood adipokines and birth size: the Hokkaido Study on environment and children's health. Environ Res. 2017;156:175–82. https://doi.org/10.1016/j.envres.2017.03.033.
27. Minatoya M, Araki A, Miyashita C, et al. Prenatal di-2-ethylhexyl phthalate exposure and cord blood adipokine levels and birth size: the Hokkaido study on environment and children's health. Sci Total Environ. 2017;579:606–11. https://doi.org/10.1016/j.scitotenv.2016.11.051.
28. Goudarzi H, Araki A, Itoh S, Sasaki S, Miyashita C, Mitsui T, Nakazawa H, Nonomura K, Kishi R. The association of prenatal exposure to perfluorinated chemicals with glucocorticoid and androgenic hormones in cord blood samples: the Hokkaido Study. Environ Health Perspect. 2017;125(1):111–8. https://doi.org/10.1289/EHP142.
29. Itoh S, Araki A, Mitsui T, et al. Association of perfluoroalkyl substances exposure in utero with reproductive hormone levels in cord blood in the Hokkaido Study on Environment and Children's Health. Environ Int. 2016;94:51–9. https://doi.org/10.1016/j.envint.2016.05.011.
30. Okada E, Kashino I, Matsuura H, et al. Temporal trends of perfluoroalkyl acids in plasma samples of pregnant women in Hokkaido, Japan, 2003-2011. Environ Int. 2013;60:89–96. https://doi.org/10.1016/j.envint.2013.07.013.
31. Yila TA, Sasaki S, Miyashita C, et al. Effects of maternal 5,10-methylenetetrahydrofolate reductase C677T and A1298C Polymorphisms and tobacco smoking on infant birth weight in a Japanese population. J Epidemiol. 2012;22(2):91–102.
32. Yamada T, Morikawa M, Yamada T, et al. First-trimester serum folate levels and subsequent risk of abortion and preterm birth among Japanese women with singleton pregnancies. Arch Gynecol Obstet. 2013;287(1):9–14. https://doi.org/10.1007/s00404-012-2501-5.
33. Sasaki S, Kondo T, Sata F, et al. Maternal smoking during pregnancy and genetic polymorphisms in the Ah receptor, CYP1A1 and GSTM1 affect infant birth size in Japanese subjects. Mol Hum Reprod. 2006;12(2):77–83. https://doi.org/10.1093/molehr/gal013.
34. Spurgeon SL, Jones RC, Ramakrishnan R. High throughput gene expression measurement with real time PCR in a microfluidic dynamic array. PLoS One. 2008;3(2):e1662. https://doi.org/10.1371/journal.pone.0001662.
35. Wang B, Tan HW, Fang W, et al. Developing single nucleotide polymorphism (SNP) markers from transcriptome sequences for identification of longan (Dimocarpus longan) germplasm. Hortic Res. 2015;2:14065. https://doi.org/10.1038/hortres.2014.65.

36. Wang J, Lin M, Crenshaw A, et al. High-throughput single nucleotide polymorphism genotyping using nanofluidic Dynamic Arrays. BMC Genomics. 2009;10:561. https://doi.org/10.1186/1471-2164-10-561.
37. Kobayashi S, Azumi K, Goudarzi H, et al. Effects of prenatal perfluoroalkyl acid exposure on cord blood IGF2/H19 methylation and ponderal index: the Hokkaido Study. J Expo Sci Environ Epidemiol. 2016; https://doi.org/10.1038/jes.2016.50.
38. Bibikova M, Barnes B, Tsan C, et al. High density DNA methylation array with single CpG site resolution. Genomics. 2011;98(4):288–95. https://doi.org/10.1016/j.ygeno.2011.07.007.
39. Sandoval J, Heyn H, Moran S, et al. Validation of a DNA methylation microarray for 450,000 CpG sites in the human genome. Epigenetics. 2011;6(6):692–702.
40. Itabashi K, Fujimura M, Kusuda S, et al. The introduction of new standard values of birth weight according to gestational age (in Japanese). J Jpn Pediatr Soc. 2010;114:1271–93.
41. Miyashita C, Sasaki S, Ikeno T, et al. Effects of in utero exposure to polychlorinated biphenyls, methylmercury, and polyunsaturated fatty acids on birth size. Sci Total Environ. 2015;533:256–65. https://doi.org/10.1016/j.scitotenv.2015.06.108.
42. Minatoya M, Nakajima S, Sasaki S, et al. Effects of prenatal phthalate exposure on thyroid hormone levels, mental and psychomotor development of infants: the Hokkaido Study on Environment and Children's Health. Sci Total Environ. 2016;565:1037–43. https://doi.org/10.1016/j.scitotenv.2016.05.098.
43. Minatoya M, Sasaki S, Araki A, et al. Cord blood bisphenol A levels and reproductive and thyroid hormone levels of neonates: the Hokkaido Study on Environment and Children's Health. Epidemiology. 2017;28 Suppl 1:S3–9. https://doi.org/10.1097/EDE.0000000000000716.
44. Braun T, Challis JR, Newnham JP, et al. Early-life glucocorticoid exposure: the hypothalamic-pituitary-adrenal axis, placental function, and long-term disease risk. Endocr Rev. 2013;34(6):885–916. https://doi.org/10.1210/er.2013-1012.
45. Reynolds RM. Corticosteroid-mediated programming and the pathogenesis of obesity and diabetes. J Steroid Biochem Mol Biol. 2010;122(1–3):3–9. https://doi.org/10.1016/j.jsbmb.2010.01.009.
46. Labrie F, Luu-The V, Labrie C, et al. DHEA and its transformation into androgens and estrogens in peripheral target tissues: intracrinology. Front Neuroendocrinol. 2001;22(3):185–212. https://doi.org/10.1006/frne.2001.0216.
47. Araki A, Mitsui T, Goudarzi H, et al. Prenatal di(2-ethylhexyl) phthalate exposure and disruption of adrenal androgens and glucocorticoids levels in cord blood: the Hokkaido Study. Sci Total Environ. 2016;581-582:297–304. https://doi.org/10.1016/j.scitotenv.2016.12.124.
48. Goudarzi H, Nakajima S, Ikeno T, et al. Prenatal exposure to perfluorinated chemicals and neurodevelopment in early infancy: the Hokkaido Study. Sci Total Environ. 2016;541:1002–10. https://doi.org/10.1016/j.scitotenv.2015.10.017.
49. Nakajima S, Saijo Y, Kato S, et al. Effects of prenatal exposure to polychlorinated biphenyls and dioxins on mental and motor development in Japanese children at 6 months of age. Environ Health Perspect. 2006;114(5):773–8.
50. Goodman R. The Strengths and Difficulties Questionnaire: a research note. J Child Psychol Psychiatry. 1997;38(5):581–6.
51. Goodman R. Psychometric properties of the strengths and difficulties questionnaire. J Am Acad Child Adolesc Psychiatry. 2001;40(11):1337–45. https://doi.org/10.1097/00004583-200111000-00015.
52. Minatoya M, Itoh S, Araki A, et al. Associated factors of behavioural problems in children at preschool age: the Hokkaido study on environment and children's health. Child Care Health Dev. 2017;43(3):385–92. https://doi.org/10.1111/cch.12424.
53. Miyashita C, Sasaki S, Saijo Y, et al. Effects of prenatal exposure to dioxin-like compounds on allergies and infections during infancy. Environ Res. 2011;111(4):551–8. https://doi.org/10.1016/j.envres.2011.01.021.
54. Goudarzi H, Miyashita C, Okada E, et al. Effects of prenatal exposure to perfluoroalkyl acids on prevalence of allergic diseases among 4-year-old children. Environ Int. 2016;94:124–32. https://doi.org/10.1016/j.envint.2016.05.020.

55. Okada E, Sasaki S, Kashino I, et al. Prenatal exposure to perfluoroalkyl acids and allergic diseases in early childhood. Environ Int. 2014;65:127–34. https://doi.org/10.1016/j.envint.2014.01.007.
56. Goudarzi H, Miyashita C, Okada E, et al. Prenatal exposure to perfluoroalkyl acids and prevalence of infectious diseases up to 4 years of age. Environ Int. 2017;104:132–8. https://doi.org/10.1016/j.envint.2017.01.024.
57. Sasaki S, Sata F, Katoh S, et al. Adverse birth outcomes associated with maternal smoking and polymorphisms in the N-Nitrosamine-metabolizing enzyme genes NQO1 and CYP2E1. Am J Epidemiol. 2008;167(6):719–26. https://doi.org/10.1093/aje/kwm360.
58. Kobayashi S, Sata F, Sasaki S, et al. Combined effects of AHR, CYP1A1, and XRCC1 genotypes and prenatal maternal smoking on infant birth size: biomarker assessment in the Hokkaido Study. Reprod Toxicol. 2016;65:295–306. https://doi.org/10.1016/j.reprotox.2016.08.020.
59. Kobayashi S, Sata F, Sasaki S, et al. Genetic association of aromatic hydrocarbon receptor (AHR) and cytochrome P450, family 1, subfamily A, polypeptide 1 (CYP1A1) polymorphisms with dioxin blood concentrations among pregnant Japanese women. Toxicol Lett. 2013;219(3):269–78. https://doi.org/10.1016/j.toxlet.2013.03.013.
60. Kobayashi S, Sata F, Miyashita C, et al. Dioxin-metabolizing genes in relation to effects of prenatal dioxin levels and reduced birth size: the Hokkaido study. Reprod Toxicol. 2017;67:111–6. https://doi.org/10.1016/j.reprotox.2016.12.002.
61. Hayes AF. Introduction to mediation, moderation, and conditional process analysis: a regression-based approach. New York, NY: Guilford Press; 2013.
62. Preacher KJ, Hayes AF. Asymptotic and resampling strategies for assessing and comparing indirect effects in multiple mediator models. Behav Res Methods. 2008;40(3):879–91.
63. Fairchild AJ, Mackinnon DP, Taborga MP, et al. R2 effect-size measures for mediation analysis. Behav Res Methods. 2009;41(2):486–98. https://doi.org/10.3758/BRM.41.2.486.
64. Kishi R, Zhang J, Ha E, et al. Birth Cohort Consortium of Asia (BiCCA) – current and future perspectives. Epidemiology. 2017;28 Suppl 1:S19–34. https://doi.org/10.1097/EDE.0000000000000698.

Chapter 10
Current Findings in a Birth Cohort Study with Omics Analysis: Chiba Study of Mother and Child Health (C-MACH)

Kenichi Sakurai and Chisato Mori

Abstract Recent epidemiological studies have shown that environmental factors like maternal nutrition, smoking habits, and economic stability during the period from pregnancy to early childhood might affect the risk of noncommunicable diseases in adulthood. This concept is referred to as "developmental origins of health and disease (DOHaD)." Exposure to chemicals is also an important risk factor for fetal development. Moreover, there is some concern that certain chemicals can affect human reproduction and development because of their endocrine-disrupting properties, especially during fetal period.

The Chiba Study of Mother and Children's Health (C-MACH) is a birth cohort study that has been conducted since 2014. The study is focused on the health effects of environmental factors (including chemicals) on fetuses and includes omics analysis to identify potential biomarkers and clarify these mechanisms.

In this article, we introduce the current findings of C-MACH, which aims to develop advanced preventive medical and strategic interventions during the fetal period that will help to lower the risk of chronic disease.

Keywords Birth cohort · Omics analysis · DOHaD · Environmental chemicals

K. Sakurai
Center for Preventive Medical Sciences, Chiba University, Chiba, Japan
e-mail: sakuraik@faculty.chiba-u.jp

C. Mori (✉)
Center for Preventive Medical Sciences, Chiba University, Chiba, Japan

Department of Bioenvironmental Medicine, Graduate School of Medicine, Chiba University, Chiba, Japan
e-mail: cmori@faculty.chiba-u.jp

F. Sata et al. (eds.), *Pre-emptive Medicine: Public Health Aspects of Developmental Origins of Health and Disease*, Current Topics in Environmental Health and Preventive Medicine, https://doi.org/10.1007/978-981-13-2194-8_10

Abbreviations

BMI	Body mass index
DOHaD	Developmental origins of health and disease
HRM analysis	High-resolution melting analysis
ISO	International Organization for Standardization
NCD	Noncommunicable disease
PCB	Polychlorinated biphenyl
POPs	Persistent organic pollutants

10.1 Introduction

There are growing global concerns about infant, child, and adolescent health, with the increasing prevalence of noncommunicable diseases (NCDs) such as obesity and diabetes, neurodevelopmental disorders, allergies and respiratory diseases, and some cancers [1–3]. In previous studies, we have reported that environmental contaminants, such as polychlorinated biphenyls (PCBs), were detected in maternal blood, umbilical cords, and cord blood [4–6]. The early stages of human development are particularly sensitive to the effects of toxicants, which can interact with the processes of developmental plasticity. Recent epidemiological studies have shown that environmental factors during the fetal period and into early childhood might affect the risk of NCDs in adulthood [7–9]. If exposure can be prevented by scientific efforts, adverse effects on the health of future generations can also be prevented.

A cohort study is an epidemiological method that tracks groups of people with or without factors of interest, to clarify the relationship between those factors and outcomes. A cohort study that starts during pregnancy is called a birth cohort study. Well-designed, large-scale birth cohort studies will lead to improved understanding that can help to prevent possible adverse effects of environmental factors, such as chemical exposure, on infant, child, and adult health.

Recently, dramatic changes in social and living environments have led to an increase in NCDs. Epidemiological research focused in European countries [7–9] has revealed the effects of the nutritional environment from the fetal period to early childhood on NCDs in adulthood. The concept of developmental origins of health and disease (DOHaD) has been proposed [7, 10], which states that the risk of a variety of chronic diseases is affected by pre- and postnatal environmental factors such as maternal nutrition during the fetal period, lifestyle, stress, and exposure to environmental pollutants, as well as genetic sensitivity. Therefore, cohort studies are required to elucidate the effects of the fetal environment, including chemical exposure, on post-birth health issues [11].

Several mechanisms of the DOHaD concept have been proposed. One of these mechanisms is epigenetic changes to the genome caused by exposure to environmental factors during the fetal period and early childhood [10]; another is changes in the gut microbiota of children, which might be affected by that of their mothers and the postnatal environment. Disruption of the gut microbiota balance (known as dysbiosis) affects the development not only of digestive system-related diseases but also of systemic conditions [12].

To evaluate these issues, omics analyses have been conducted in recent years. Epigenomic analysis, such as *epigenome*-wide association studies (EWAS), is applied to assess epigenetic changes; metagenomic analyses, such as 16S rRNA gene amplicon sequencing analysis, are used to assess gut microbiota. Additionally, metabolomic analysis, the exhaustive analysis of in vivo metabolites, has provided a more detailed understanding of changes occurring in vivo. Thus, the effects of environmental factors on health as well as the underlying mechanisms can be evaluated using these omics analyses.

A limited number of epidemiological studies have comprehensively used these novel analytical techniques and concepts. The analyses of epigenetic changes, gut microbiota, and the metabolome in epidemiological research might help to identify new biomarkers for predicting disease risk and determining the effects of environmental factors at an early stage.

In this article, we introduce the current findings of our cohort study, the Chiba Study of Mother and Children's Health (C-MACH), obtained using new research techniques such as omics, with the aim to develop advanced preventive medical and strategic interventions during the fetal period that will help to lower the risk of chronic disease.

10.2 About C-MACH

The C-MACH study was planned as a birth cohort study using omics analysis, including genome analysis, in addition to the aforementioned analyses to evaluate the effects of fetal and early childhood environmental factors on children's health [13]. C-MACH began in 2014 and is currently underway. The study consists of three hospital-based cohorts from Onodera Ladies Clinic and Yamaguchi Women's Hospital, both in Chiba Prefecture, Japan, and Aiwa Hospital in Saitama Prefecture.

The purpose of this study is to explore the effects of genetic and environmental factors, particularly the fetal environment and post-birth living environment, on children's health, and to identify biomarkers for these effects (Fig. 10.1). Primary outcomes of C-MACH are allergies, obesity, endocrine and metabolic disorders, and developmental disorders.

The following are our specific, approved research objectives:

1. Ascertain the links between nutritional intake by pregnant women and fetal development.
2. Establish biomarkers and indicators of epigenetic alteration to predict children's health problems, such as obesity, allergies, and impaired mental development.
3. Ascertain whether the interaction between fetal/neonatal environmental factors and genotypes is associated with mental development during childhood.

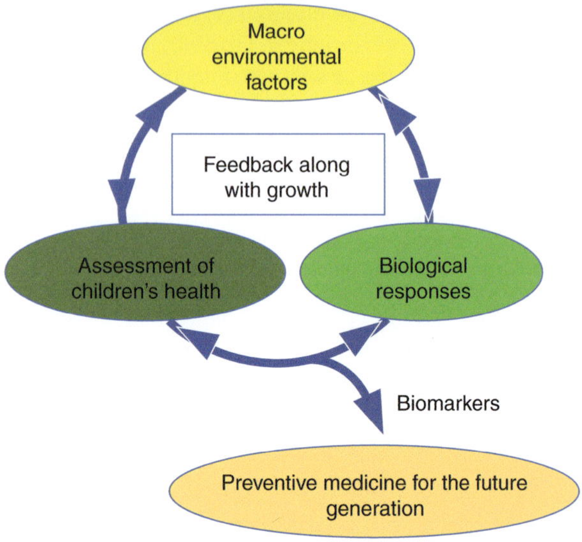

Fig. 10.1 Purpose and strategy of C-MACH

4. Ascertain whether the gut microbiota of mothers affects the development and health of their children, and clarify the factors that affect post-birth changes in gut microbiota.
5. Ascertain the effects of fetal exposure to environmental chemicals on epigenetic changes or the blood metabolome in children.

Pregnant women at less than 13 weeks' gestation were recruited. During pregnancy, participants underwent normal monitoring at the three hospitals. In the event of a stillbirth, participation in the cohort ceased for the mother. The recruitment population also consisted of all children born to women who consented to participate. The fathers of all recruited children were also candidates for participation. Participating women are withdrawn from the study if they are transferred to a different hospital for any reason.

Recruitment began in February 2014 and ended in June 2015. All participants provided written consent including completing questionnaire surveys and the collection, storage, and analyses of biological and home environmental samples.

All participants will be followed until the child reaches the age of 5 years. Follow-up will mainly be completed via questionnaire. Follow-up after the age of 5 years will be considered later.

During the first and last trimesters, questionnaires were administered, and blood, urine, and feces samples were collected. The questionnaire items include socioeconomic status, lifestyle habits, a brief diet history questionnaire, and psychological assessment.

We collected the usual medical findings at birth as well as umbilical cords, umbilical cord blood, placenta, and fecal samples. Data for the children are collected from health checkup records and questionnaires about child development and disease history at the ages of 1 month, 4 months, 10 months, 1.5 years, 3.5 years, and 5 years.

All biological samples are stored at −80 °C in the Chiba University Center for Preventive Medical Sciences BioBank. They will be preserved as biological specimens until the analysis is completed.

Until now, 434 women have provided their written consent to participate in C-MACH; 68 women withdrew after providing informed consent; as a result, 366 women are currently participating. We collected and analyzed questionnaires from 376 women in the early gestational period. The mean age of 376 participants was 32.5 (±4.4) years, and the mean age of women expecting their first child was 31.8 (±4.2) years. This was older than the mean age of the Japanese population (29.7 years) [14]. A total 98.4% of women were married, and 72.3% had an appropriate prepregnancy BMI (18.5–24.9 kg/m^2). Smokers during early pregnancy accounted for 5.0% of participants, which is lower than the percentage in other Japanese cohort studies [15–17].

10.3 Multilevel Analysis: Omics and Exposure

Omics analysis is a comprehensive method for analyzing various biological phenomena and includes several methodological approaches. Genomics targets genetic information, transcriptomics targets mRNA, and proteomics targets protein. Additionally, epigenetic alterations, metabolic changes, and microbiota are becoming target omics research fields; the analyses in these interesting fields are called epigenomics, metabolomics, and metagenomics, respectively. These comprehensive methods enable greater understanding of the mechanisms or risks of various diseases, to establish more precise medical approaches in the future.

Recently, these omics analyses are being performed in birth cohort studies, such as the Human Early-Life Exposome (HELIX) study and Tohoku Medical Megabank Project, among others [18, 19]. The DOHaD hypothesis proposes that interaction between genetic and environmental factors contributes to the onset of NCDs. Thus, it is useful to perform omics analyses in a birth cohort study, to detect the changes that appear before the onset of NCDs. Particularly, omics analyses targeting mothers, fetuses, and infants are important because of the fragility and plasticity of the fetus and infant.

In the C-MACH study, we plan to perform several omics analyses (Fig. 10.2): genomics, epigenomics, metabolomics, and metagenomics. Epigenetic changes, such as DNA methylation, are known to persist for a long period, thereby affecting human health and disease in adulthood.

10.3.1 Epigenetic Analysis

DNA methylation is one of the mechanisms hypothesized in the DOHaD model [20]. Comprehensive epigenetic analyses to investigate DNA methylation in the umbilical cord have been reported [21], with the use of a microarray (Illumina iScan system and Infinium HumanMethylation450 BeadChip, Illumina, San Diego, CA, USA) and methylation-sensitive high-resolution melting (HRM) analysis [22, 23]. In C-MACH, we are examining variations in the DNA methylation of umbilical

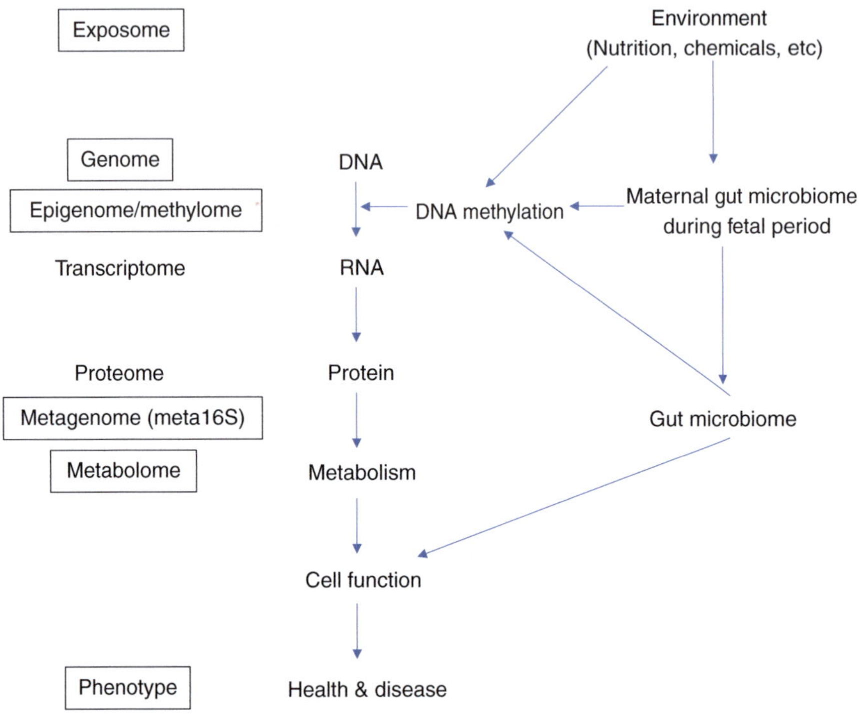

Fig. 10.2 The multilevel analysis of C-MACH. The analyses planned in C-MACH are indicated by solid lines

cords using a DNA methylation array. We will extract CpG sites that are correlated with outcomes, and detected candidate areas will be examined using HRM or pyrosequencing for all umbilical cord samples.

We performed pilot analysis to explore the relationship between umbilical cord DNA methylation and maternal factors. We found that DNA methylation of the umbilical cord at several CpG sites assessed by HRM or methylation array is associated with maternal factors. In one of these sites, methylation levels of the *H19* gene were associated with the mother's age [24]. The methylation levels of this gene may be regulated or affected by maternal aging, and it may cause some health effects in their children as this gene is important for fetal growth [25].

10.3.2 Metagenomic Analysis

The gut microbiome has come to be considered a novel environmental factor that affects our health [26–28]. Perturbations in the gut microbiome have been implicated in the cause of metabolic syndrome [29], and the role of the gut microbiome in pregnancy has become the subject of considerable interest [30].

Gut microbiota is analyzed using 16S rRNA gene sequences [31] or whole metagenomic sequences. In C-MACH, the DNA of gut microbiota is extracted from stool samples collected from mothers and their children, and we are analyzing the distribution and bias of gut microbiota using 16S rRNA sequence data.

We conducted a pilot study using maternal gut microbiota data. We did not detect any significant correlation between the proportion of the phylum *Firmicutes* and maternal anthropometric or nutritional parameters, such as maternal prepregnancy BMI, body weight gain during pregnancy, or caloric intake; however, these results might be owing to the small sample size. We then performed analysis combining maternal gut microbiota and epigenetic data. Surprisingly, a significant correlation between *Firmicutes* phylum of maternal gut microbiota and DNA methylation of CpG sites in diabetes-associated genes was found [31]. We are currently conducting this analysis using a larger sample size.

10.3.3 Metabolomic Analysis

Metabolome analyses have been used in toxicological and epidemiological studies to provide information about the biochemical status of a biological system [32]. Metabolome analysis can provide valuable insights relating to the biological responses to environmental changes [33, 34]. The composition of metabolites, such as amino acids, lipid metabolites, and vitamins in blood and urine, is analyzed using high-performance liquid chromatography/tandem mass spectrometry [35]. We are searching for biomarkers that reflect environmental exposure and studying the mechanisms for changes in metabolomes.

We reported our first results of metabolomic analysis in association with PCB concentrations. Citraconic acid in maternal serum and ethanolamine, *p*-hydroxybenzoate, and purine in cord serum were significant in the prediction model for classification of low versus high PCB concentration groups. There are several candidate biomarkers and metabolites included in composited models relating to glutathione and amino acid metabolism in maternal serum and compounds related to amino acid metabolism and ubiquinone and other terpenoid-quinone biosyntheses in cord serum [6].

10.3.4 Genomic Analysis

In the C-MACH study, genomic analysis will be conducted using maternal blood samples and saliva samples from participating children and partners. DNA will be extracted, and genome-wide association analysis using single-nucleotide polymorphisms will be performed to examine the genomic effects on outcomes, such as allergies.

10.3.5 Environmental Chemicals

We are assessing PCB levels in maternal and umbilical cord blood as an index of the exposure to persistent organic pollutants (POPs). We previously reported that PCB concentrations in blood and umbilical cord samples are correlated with the concentrations of various POPs [4, 5, 36–39]. Additionally, indoor dust samples have been collected and will be measured for house dust, mites, mold, and endotoxins to assess the effects of the indoor environment.

PCB levels are measured using gas chromatography-mass spectrometry [40, 41]. We have obtained International Organization for Standardization (ISO) laboratory certification for blood PCB measurement. In addition to total concentration, the composition of major individual congeners is assessed and the source of exposure inferred.

We reported that the association between diet habit and serum PCB concentration was assessed in our ISO-accredited laboratory. Interestingly, cooking methods were associated with serum PCB concentration in addition to foodstuffs [42]. Recently, we proposed new life course intervention including a virtuous cycle for reducing exposure to POPs for a healthier future [43].

10.4 Future Prospects and Conclusion

In this paper, we reviewed the profile and current findings of our birth cohort study with omics techniques, C-MACH. With the valuable results obtained from omics analysis of study participants' exposome, epigenome, microbiome, and metabolome, it may be possible to identify relationships between previously unknown social or environmental factors, such as certain pollutants and health risks. As a result of our birth cohort study, we hope that adverse health effects can be reduced to contribute to healthier future generations. Our mission and that of the current generation is to decrease adverse environmental effects so as to create a better living environment for all.

References

1. Global status report on noncommunicable diseases 2010. Geneva: World Health Organization; 2011. http://www.who.int/nmh/publications/ncd_report_full_en.pdf.
2. Prevention of allergy and allergic asthma. Geneva: World Health Organization; 2003. http://www.who.int/respiratory/publications/allergy_prevention/en/.
3. Mental health and development. Geneva: World Health Organization; 2010. http://apps.who.int/iris/bitstream/10665/44257/1/9789241563949_eng.pdf.
4. Fukata H, Omori M, Osada H, Todaka E, Mori C. Necessity to measure PCBs and organochlorine pesticide concentrations in human umbilical cords for fetal exposure assessment. Environ Health Perspect. 2005;113(3):297–303.

5. Ochiai S, Shimojo N, Yuka I, Watanabe M, Matsuno Y, Suzuki S, et al. A pilot study for foetal exposure to multiple persistent organic pollutants and the development of infant atopic dermatitis in modern Japanese society. Chemosphere. 2014;94:48–52.
6. Eguchi A, Sakurai K, Watanabe M, Mori C. Exploration of potential biomarkers and related biological pathways for PCB exposure in maternal and cord serum: a pilot birth cohort study in Chiba. Jpn Environ Int. 2017;102:157–64.
7. Barker DJ, Winter PD, Osmond C, Margetts B, Simmonds SJ. Weight in infancy and death from ischaemic heart disease. Lancet. 1989;2(8663):577–80.
8. Roseboom T, de Rooij S, Painter R. The Dutch famine and its long-term consequences for adult health. Early Hum Dev. 2006;82(8):485–91.
9. Stein AD, Zybert PA, van der Pal-de Bruin K, Lumey LH. Exposure to famine during gestation, size at birth, and blood pressure at age 59 y: evidence from the Dutch Famine. Eur J Epidemiol. 2006;21(10):759–65.
10. Gluckman PD, Hanson MA. Living with the past: evolution, development, and patterns of disease. Science. 2004;305(5691):1733–6.
11. Gehring U, Casas M, Brunekreef B, Bergstrom A, Bonde JP, Botton J, et al. Environmental exposure assessment in European birth cohorts: results from the ENRIECO project. Environ Health. 2013;12:8.
12. Le Chatelier E, Nielsen T, Qin J, Prifti E, Hildebrand F, Falony G, et al. Richness of human gut microbiome correlates with metabolic markers. Nature. 2013;500(7464):541–6.
13. Sakurai K, Miyaso H, Eguchi A, Matsuno Y, Yamamoto M, Todaka E, et al. Chiba study of Mother and Children's Health (C-MACH): cohort study with omics analyses. BMJ Open. 2016;6(1):e010531.
14. Ministry of Health, Labour and Welfare. Specified report of vital statistics in FY2010. Tokyo, Japan; 2010. http://www.mhlw.go.jp/english/database/db-hw/FY2010/live_births.html.
15. Suzuki K, Tanaka T, Kondo N, Minai J, Sato M, Yamagata Z. Is maternal smoking during early pregnancy a risk factor for all low birth weight infants? J Epidemiol. 2008;18(3):89–96.
16. Michikawa T, Nitta H, Nakayama SF, Ono M, Yonemoto J, Tamura K, et al. The Japan Environment and Children's Study (JECS): a preliminary report on selected characteristics of approximately 10 000 pregnant women recruited during the first year of the study. J Epidemiol. 2015;25(6):452–8.
17. Otake Y, Nakajima S, Uno A, Kato S, Sasaki S, Yoshioka E, et al. Association between maternal antenatal depression and infant development: a hospital-based prospective cohort study. Environ Health Prev Med. 2014;19(1):30–45.
18. Kuriyama S, Yaegashi N, Nagami F, Arai T, Kawaguchi Y, Osumi N, et al. The Tohoku medical megabank project: design and mission. J Epidemiol. 2016;26(9):493–511.
19. Vrijheid M, Slama R, Robinson O, Chatzi L, Coen M, van den Hazel P, et al. The human early-life exposome (HELIX): project rationale and design. Environ Health Perspect. 2014;122(6):535–44.
20. Kupers LK, Xu X, Jankipersadsing SA, Vaez A, la Bastide-van Gemert S, Scholtens S, et al. DNA methylation mediates the effect of maternal smoking during pregnancy on birthweight of the offspring. Int J Epidemiol. 2015;44(4):1224–37.
21. Tse MY, Ashbury JE, Zwingerman N, King WD, Taylor SA, Pang SC. A refined, rapid and reproducible high resolution melt (HRM)-based method suitable for quantification of global LINE-1 repetitive element methylation. BMC Res Notes. 2011;4:565.
22. Gao WL, Li D, Xiao ZX, Liao QP, Yang HX, Li YX, et al. Detection of global DNA methylation and paternally imprinted H19 gene methylation in preeclamptic placentas. Hypertens Res. 2011;34(5):655–61.
23. Wojdacz TK, Dobrovic A, Algar EM. Rapid detection of methylation change at H19 in human imprinting disorders using methylation-sensitive high-resolution melting. Hum Mutat. 2008;29(10):1255–60.
24. Miyaso H, Sakurai K, Takase S, Eguchi A, Watanabe M, Fukuoka H, et al. The methylation levels of the H19 differentially methylated region in human umbilical cords reflect newborn

parameters and changes by maternal environmental factors during early pregnancy. Environ Res. 2017;157:1–8.
25. Kitsiou-Tzeli S, Tzetis M. Maternal epigenetics and fetal and neonatal growth. Curr Opin Endocrinol Diabetes Obes. 2017;24(1):43–6.
26. Subramanian S, Blanton LV, Frese SA, Charbonneau M, Mills DA, Gordon JI. Cultivating healthy growth and nutrition through the gut microbiota. Cell. 2015;161(1):36–48.
27. Bisgaard H, Li N, Bonnelykke K, Chawes BL, Skov T, Paludan-Muller G, et al. Reduced diversity of the intestinal microbiota during infancy is associated with increased risk of allergic disease at school age. J Allergy Clin Immunol. 2011;128(3):646–52.e1–5.
28. Pfefferle PI, Prescott SL, Kopp M. Microbial influence on tolerance and opportunities for intervention with prebiotics/probiotics and bacterial lysates. J Allergy Clin Immunol. 2013;131(6):1453–63; quiz 64.
29. Ley RE, Backhed F, Turnbaugh P, Lozupone CA, Knight RD, Gordon JI. Obesity alters gut microbial ecology. Proc Natl Acad Sci U S A. 2005;102(31):11070–5.
30. Koren O, Goodrich JK, Cullender TC, Spor A, Laitinen K, Backhed HK, et al. Host remodeling of the gut microbiome and metabolic changes during pregnancy. Cell. 2012;150(3):470–80.
31. Tachibana K, Sakurai K, Watanabe M, Miyaso H, Mori C. Associations between changes in the maternal gut microbiome and differentially methylated regions of diabetes-associated genes in fetuses: a pilot study from a birth cohort study. J Diabetes Investig. 2017;8(4):550–3.
32. Fearnley LG, Inouye M. Metabolomics in epidemiology: from metabolite concentrations to integrative reaction networks. Int J Epidemiol. 2016;45(5):1319–28.
33. Robertson DG, Watkins PB, Reily MD. Metabolomics in toxicology: preclinical and clinical applications. Toxicol Sci. 2011;120(Suppl 1):S146–70.
34. Ramirez T, Daneshian M, Kamp H, Bois FY, Clench MR, Coen M, et al. Metabolomics in toxicology and preclinical research. ALTEX. 2013;30(2):209–25.
35. Yuan M, Breitkopf SB, Yang X, Asara JM. A positive/negative ion-switching, targeted mass spectrometry-based metabolomics platform for bodily fluids, cells, and fresh and fixed tissue. Nat Protoc. 2012;7(5):872–81.
36. Mori C, Fukata H, Sakurai K, Jotaki T, Todaka E, Saito Y. Strong correlation between the concentration of dioxins and total PCBs in current Japanese people. Chemosphere. 2008;73(1 Suppl):S235–8.
37. Mori C, Komiyama M, Adachi T, Sakurai K, Nishimura D, Takashima K, et al. Application of toxicogenomic analysis to risk assessment of delayed long-term effects of multiple chemicals, including endocrine disruptors in human fetuses. EHP Toxicogenomics. 2003;111(1T):7–13.
38. Mori C, Kakuta K, Matsuno Y, Todaka E, Watanabe M, Hanazato M, et al. Polychlorinated biphenyl levels in the blood of Japanese individuals ranging from infants to over 80 years of age. Environ Sci Pollut Res Int. 2014;21(10):6434–9.
39. Mori C, Nakamura N, Todaka E, Fujisaki T, Matsuno Y, Nakaoka H, et al. Correlation between human maternal-fetal placental transfer and molecular weight of PCB and dioxin congeners/isomers. Chemosphere. 2014;114:262–7.
40. Sjodin A, Jones RS, Lapeza CR, Focant JF, McGahee EE 3rd, Patterson DG Jr. Semiautomated high-throughput extraction and cleanup method for the measurement of polybrominated diphenyl ethers, polybrominated biphenyls, and polychlorinated biphenyls in human serum. Anal Chem. 2004;76(7):1921–7.
41. Flores-Ramirez R, Ortiz-Perez MD, Batres-Esquivel L, Castillo CG, Ilizaliturri-Hernandez CA, Diaz-Barriga F. Rapid analysis of persistent organic pollutants by solid phase microextraction in serum samples. Talanta. 2014;123:169–78.
42. Jin W, Otake M, Eguchi A, Sakurai K, Nakaoka H, Watanabe M, et al. Dietary habits and cooking methods could reduce avoidable exposure to PCBs in maternal and cord sera. Sci Rep. 2017;7(1):17357.
43. Mori C, Todaka E. For a healthier future: a virtuous cycle for reducing exposure to persistent organic pollutants. J Epidemiol Community Health. 2017;71(7):660–2.

Chapter 11
Neurodevelopmental Disorders in the Hamamatsu Birth Cohort for Mothers and Children (HBC Study)

Kenji J. Tsuchiya and Shu Takagai

The HBC Study team, including past members, are (in an alphabetical order): Ms. Sanae Aoyagi, Rie Gonda, Emi Hatano, Emi Higashimoto, Maiko Honda, Tomoyo Isobe, Noriko Kodera, Yumeno Kugizaki, Hiroko Muraki, Atsuko Nakamura, Chikako Nakayasu, Makiko Narumiya, Yuko Nishimura, Michiyo Nishizawa, Yuko Osuka, Eriko Sato, Haruka Suzuki, Yukiko Suzuki, Riyo Takabayashi, Mana Yamashita, Mr. Ryuji Nakahara, Kei Shigeno, Drs. Ryosuke Asano, Damee Choi, Yusaku Endoh, Taeko Harada, Koichi Hirano, Takanobu Horikoshi, Thanseem Ismail, Hiroaki Itoh, Toshiki Iwabuchi, Keiko Iwata, Yasuhide Iwata, Yosuke Kameno, Naohiro Kanayama, Emiko Kawai, Masayoshi Kawai, Daisuke Kurita, Yujin K. Kuroda, Hitoshi Kuwabara, Kaori Matsumoto, Taishi Miyachi, Hideo Matsuzaki, Norio Mori, Tsuruko Mori, Kyoko Nakaizumi, Kazuhiko Nakamura, Tomoko Nishimura, Yoko Nomura, Ryuichiro Ohshima, Akemi Okumura, Anitha A. Pillai, Yoko Sagawa, Chie Shimmura, Yui Seno, Shiro Suda, Genichi Sugihara, Katsuaki Suzuki, Teruhiko Suzuki, Kiyokazu Takebayashi, Nori Takei, Masatsugu Tsujii, Satoshi Uchiyama, Mahesh Mundalil Vasu, Tomoyasu Wakuda, Keisuke Wakusawa, Manabu Wakuta, Kohei Yamada, Hidenori Yamasue and Masamichi Yokokura.

K. J. Tsuchiya (✉)
Research Center for Child Mental Development, Hamamatsu University School of Medicine, Hamamatsu, Japan

United Graduate School of Child Development, Hamamatsu University School of Medicine, Hamamatsu, Japan
e-mail: tsuchiya@hama-med.ac.jp

S. Takagai
United Graduate School of Child Development, Hamamatsu University School of Medicine, Hamamatsu, Japan

Department of Child and Adolescent Psychiatry, Hamamatsu University School of Medicine, Hamamatsu, Japan

F. Sata et al. (eds.), *Pre-emptive Medicine: Public Health Aspects of Developmental Origins of Health and Disease*, Current Topics in Environmental Health and Preventive Medicine, https://doi.org/10.1007/978-981-13-2194-8_11

Abstract Neurodevelopmental disorders are a collective term that encompasses neuropsychiatric conditions whose manifestations occurs very early in life. Among these, attention-deficit hyperactivity disorder (ADHD) and autism spectrum disorder (ASD) are the two most common and prevalent disorders. In clinical reality, however, no single sign or symptom that is solely associated with a later diagnosis of ADHD or ASD; early trajectories that lead to ADHD or ASD remains to be investigated. In addition, growing number of studies have reported environmental risk factors for ADHD and ASD, which may account for unexplained aetiology of these disorders. To this point, researchers in this field have been keen to elucidate early trajectories and environmental risk factors for ADHD and ASD using birth cohorts based on general population. The authors established the Hamamatsu Birth Cohort for Mothers and Children (HBC Study) in 2007. A total of 1258 neonates from 1138 mothers were included and are planned to be followed up for 8 years. The HBC Study team found that five, neurodevelopmental trajectories during the first two years were extracted; three out of five trajectory classes were associated with an increased risk for having a diagnosis of ASD. The HBC Study will provide a unique and valuable resource for providing new insights into neurodevelopmental disorders.

Keywords Neurodevelopment · Attention-deficit hyperactivity disorder (ADHD) · Autism spectrum disorder (ASD) · Birth Cohort

Abbreviations

ADHD	Attention-deficit hyperactivity disorder
ADHD-RS	ADHD Rating Scale
ADOS	Autism Diagnostic Observation Schedule
ASD	Autism spectrum disorder
CI	Confidence interval
DSM-5	Diagnostic and Statistical Manual of Mental Disorders, Fifth Edition
DSM-IV	Diagnostic and Statistical Manual of Mental Disorders, Fourth Edition
HBC Study	Hamamatsu Birth Cohort for Mothers and Children
ICD-10	International Classification of Mental and Behavioural Disorders, Tenth Edition
M-CHAT	Modified Checklist for Autism in Toddlers
MSEL	Mullen Scales of Early Learning
PFOS	Perfluorooctane sulfonate
POPs	Persistent organic pollutants
SD	Standard deviation
SDQ	Strength and Difficulties Questionnaire
WISC-IV	Wechsler Intelligence Scale for Children, Fourth edition
WPPSI	Wechsler Preschool and Primary Scale of Intelligence

11.1 Neurodevelopmental Disorders in Children: What We Know

The term "neurodevelopmental disorders" encompasses a collection of medical, neuropsychiatric, and behavioural conditions whose first manifestations occur during infancy or childhood. These conditions are accompanied by impairment and/or delay in the development of functions that are closely related to biological maturation and tend to exhibit courses that do not wax and wane [1]. Specific neurodevelopmental disorders that meet these standards are described in the *International Classification of Mental and Behavioural Disorders, Tenth Edition* (ICD-10) [2], and *Diagnostic and Statistical Manual of Mental Disorders, Fifth Edition* (DSM-5) [3]. Among such specific conditions, attention-deficit hyperactivity disorder (ADHD) and autism spectrum disorder (ASD) are the two most prevalent and most commonly investigated.

ADHD is characterised by the existence of significant inattention, hyperactivity, and impulsivity [3]. The first clinical manifestation may be observed as early as during infancy, although it typically appears no later than 7 years of age [3]. The prevalence of ADHD has been reported between 5 and 10% [4, 5], although this value varies depending on the region [6–8]. This variance may stem from varying diagnostic practices as well as cultural factors [7]. Although clinical outcomes also vary [9], an increased risk for the development of conduct disorders has been well documented in patients with ADHD [10]. Research has demonstrated the efficacy of pharmacological treatment in conjunction with behavioural approaches.

ASD—which collectively refers to the conditions previously described as autism, Asperger syndrome, and pervasive developmental disorder—is characterised by impairments in social interaction and communication, in addition to repetitive behaviours and limited interests [3]. The first clinical manifestations are invariably observed during infancy, with an onset occurring by the age of 3 years [3]. The prevalence of ASD is estimated between 1 and 3% [11–15]. In spite of modest improvement after childhood reported in the literature, difficulties in social and daily life are usually long-lasting and continue throughout adulthood [16]. Successful pharmacological treatment of ASD has not been established, although various behavioural, psychological, and educational methods can be used to ameliorate a range of difficulties inherent to ASD [17].

Recent clinical, biological, and longitudinal studies have postulated that ADHD and ASD might share a common aetiology [18, 19]. Indeed, recent updates to the diagnostic criteria align with these observations [3]. Research has demonstrated that, for both ADHD and ASD, early intervention leads to better outcomes by reducing difficulties directly associated with symptoms and behavioural traits, as well as those linked to secondary depression, anxiety, and social problems [20–23].

11.2 Reported Prevalence of Neurodevelopmental Disorders of Children: Is It Increasing?

Since the 1970s, numerous studies have investigated the prevalence of ADHD, ASD, and other neurodevelopmental disorders. Notably, reported estimates for both ADHD and ASD have increased since the early 1990s in many countries [13, 14, 24, 25]. The approximately tenfold increase in the reported prevalence of ASD over the past two to three decades has become a major concern. The earliest estimates reported an ASD prevalence of approximately 1 in 1000 [26], although current, reliable estimates suggest a prevalence of approximately 1–2% [11–14]. The highest estimate (2.64%) was reported among school-age children in South Korea in 2011 [15].

Researchers have speculated that this increase in prevalence is due to changes in diagnostic criteria/practices, changes in the availability of child neuropsychiatric services, and increased awareness of neurodevelopmental disorders [24, 27]. Indeed, such explanations correspond well to the decrease in age at first diagnosis of neurodevelopmental disorders observed during the last two decades [28].

Although the precise reason for the increased prevalence of ASD remains debated, it is clear that the growing concern over these disorders has inevitably followed this trend [29]. The annual financial cost has been reported to be increased as high as 30,000 US dollars per patient [30]. In addition, the caregivers are sometimes exposed to problems associated with the condition, such as reductions in employment and leisure time [31]. Such problems are more likely to occur in the families of individuals with ASD than in those with other neurodevelopmental disorders such as ADHD [32, 33]. Of note, a delay in the first diagnosis has been associated with an increase in indirect costs to the family (e.g. additional insurance costs) [30]. These findings are likely the result of poorer clinical courses due to the lack of early intervention strategies. Therefore, early diagnosis and detection of neurodevelopmental disorders is critical in a public health context.

11.2.1 Early Diagnosis/Detection

Early diagnosis of ADHD tends to be slightly easier than early diagnosis of ASD, since the onset of ADHD is generally observable in various social and medical contexts during childhood, whereas the onset of ASD occurs during infancy, when medical examinations cannot always be conducted cooperatively. In addition, most ADHD symptoms are usually distinctive and visible, whereas ASD symptoms are sometimes occult and invisible, such as lack of typical eye contact or social awareness, which are often overlooked both by caregivers and childcare specialists [34].

A number of studies have documented that signs of ASD may appear as early as 1 year of age or even earlier [35, 36]. While some such signs have a high predictive value, there is no single sign or symptom that is solely associated with a later diagnosis of ASD. Until recently, studies have suggested that some children with

ASD may lose their diagnosis along the developmental trajectory—a phenomenon referred to as the "optimal outcome" [37, 38].

Nevertheless, many childcare specialists have successfully predicted a diagnosis of ASD in children as young as 1 year old. How is this possible? Landa and colleagues argued that certain developmental trajectory patterns, instead of a single sign, may be specific to later outcomes of ASD—a finding supported by some longitudinal and prospective studies [39–42]. These studies have provided new insight into the valid prediction of ASD during infancy; however, because the expected number of children with a diagnosis of ASD is approximately 1–2%, prospective studies in search of early trajectories specific to ASD are bound to suffer from limited statistical power. As such, previous studies have included individuals at increased risk for ASD (i.e. siblings of children with ASD). While such designs are more efficient, they do not necessarily provide useful or valid predictive methods that can be applied to the general population.

11.2.2 Environmental Risk Factors

Although both ADHD and ASD are strongly associated with genetic background [43–45], a range of risk factors that are not primarily genetic in nature have also been associated with an increased risk for these conditions. For instance, low birth weight (below 2500 g) has been reported to increase the risk of both ADHD [46, 47] and ASD [48]. However, low birth weight has a detrimental effect on child neurodevelopment in itself and thus cannot be considered a specific risk factor exclusive to these disorders [49]. Rather, suggested risk factors such as low birth weight, prematurity, and paternal age may mediate the risk of ADHD and/or ASD in individuals with a genetic predisposition for these conditions [50–52].

Environmental exposure to certain chemicals has also attracted the attention of researchers: Studies have indicated that prenatal exposure to perfluorooctane sulfonate (PFOS), persistent organic pollutants (POPs), may increase the risk of ADHD and ASD [53, 54]. Pre- and perinatal exposure to air pollution (PM2.5 and 10 in particular) have also been reported to increase the risk of ASD [55, 56]. However, such findings remain inconclusive, largely because these studies are case-control studies or high-risk cohort studies. More predictive data based on prospective cohort studies involving individuals recruited from the general population are therefore required.

11.3 HBC Study as a General-Population Cohort Study

The lack of valid prospective data based on general population for the prediction of neurodevelopmental disorders during early childhood, as well as the lack of evidence regarding the contribution of environmental/chemical exposure to the emergence of the disorders, necessitates further investigation of neurodevelopmental disorders. The

Hamamatsu Birth Cohort for Mothers and Children (HBC Study) was designed to elucidate the early developmental trajectories of children living in community settings in Japan. The major aims of the HBC study include the (1) identification of specific trajectories related to ADHD and/or ASD and the (2) identification of environmental risk factors for such trajectories.

In the following sections, we will describe how the HBC Study has been organised and provide an example of the reported findings focusing on the association between early developmental trajectories and neurodevelopmental disorders: ASD in particular.

11.3.1 Participants

The HBC Study invited all women who were in the first or second trimester of pregnancy who had visited our two research sites between November 2007 and March 2011 to participate. All women who agreed to participate in the study provided written informed consent and agreed to donate birth tissues, including cord blood, at delivery.

A total of 1408 women were invited to participate in the study (encompassing 1518 pregnancies, including 106 women who were contacted for 2 separate pregnancies and 2 women who were contacted for three separate pregnancies during the enrolment period). After the initial interviews requesting participation, the overall turnout was 82%. The remaining 1240 pregnancies (including 19 pregnancies involving twins) in 1139 women (including 99 women with two pregnancies and 1 woman with 3 pregnancies during the enrolment period) were included in the study. One pregnancy in one woman was excluded due to foetal death. The final study cohort included 1258 neonates (including 38 twins) from 1138 mothers (Fig. 11.1).

An asian custom known as *satogaeri bunben* or return-home delivery [57] is observable in our sample, in which a pregnant woman stays with her parents beginning approximately 1 month before the due date until approximately 1 month after delivery, for the purpose of receiving her parents' care. Although families who opt for *satogaeri bunben* were expected to drop out at a very early stage of follow-up, they were included in our original dataset.

The overall dropout rate for the first 2 years of the follow-up period was 16% (202/1258). However, the dropout rate following the removal of the anticipated dropouts due to *satogaeri bunben* (n = 108 infants) was 8.2% ([202–108]/[1258–108]). Importantly, the demographic and perinatal data from mothers and infants of the *satogaeri bunben* group did not differ from those of participants included in the follow-up.

11.3.2 Length of Follow-Up and Outcomes

Neurodevelopment in children was directly assessed by trained examiners at 1, 4, 6, 10, 14, 18, and 24 months. After 24 months, the children were followed up at 32 months, 40 months, 4 1/2 years, 6 years, and 8 years.

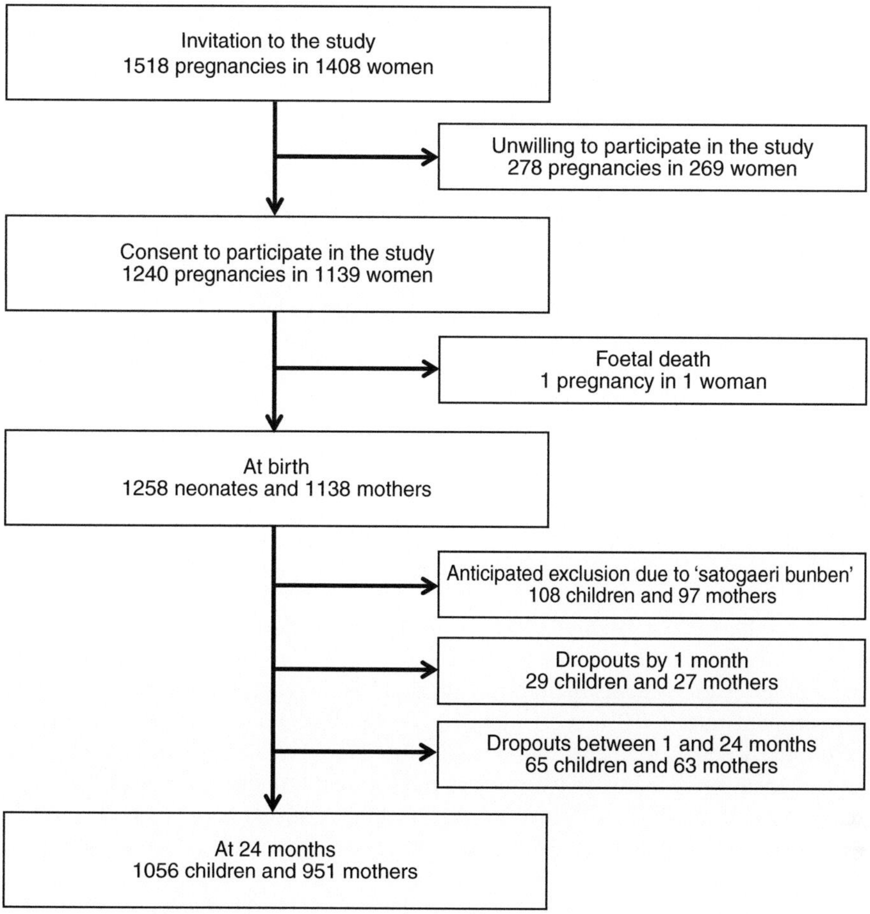

Fig. 11.1 Enrolment process and dropouts by 24 months

At the recruitment visit, questionnaires were administered to the pregnant women to capture data on demographics, socioeconomic status, lifestyle, and maternal well-being including anthropological, obstetric, medical, and psychiatric health. We specialise in collecting maternal history of psychiatric disorders using the Structured Clinical Interview for DSM-IV Axis I Disorders (SCID-I) [58].

A key feature of the HBC Study is the face-to-face assessment of neurodevelopmental status in all participating infants. At each time point between 1 and 40 months, neurodevelopment was assessed using the Mullen Scales of Early Learning (MSEL) [59]. The MSEL is a composite scale for the assessment of child development consisting of five domains: gross motor, visual reception, fine motor, receptive language, and expressive language. To assess the developmental trajectories for each of the five domains, MSEL *T*-scores, which are equivalent to *Z*-scores but with a mean of 50 and a standard deviation of 10, were generated [59].

General cognitive development was assessed at 4 1/2 years and 8 years using the Japanese version of the Wechsler Preschool and Primary Scale of Intelligence (WPPSI) [60] and the Wechsler Intelligence Scale for Children, Fourth edition (WISC-IV) [61].

The Japanese version of the Modified Checklist for Autism in Toddlers (M-CHAT) [62, 63] was used at 10, 14, or 18 months to evaluate early symptoms and signs of ASD. Furthermore, a portion of the Autism Diagnostic Observation Schedule (ADOS) [64] was adopted to evaluate qualitative abnormalities in response to joint attention at 10, 14, 18, and 24 months. At 24 months, our study team—which included a child psychiatrist and a developmental psychologist—made a clinical "red flag" judgement based on the "Practice Parameter" criteria proposed by the American Academy of Neurology and the Child Neurology Society [65]. The participating children were also evaluated for symptoms of ADHD using the SDQ at 4 1/2 and 6 years and the ADHD rating scale (ADHD-RS) [66] at 6 years. ADOS was also administered to all the children at 6 years in order to finalise whether the children had a diagnosis of ASD.

11.3.3 Strengths

The strengths of the HBC study include (1) the face-to-face assessments conducted for all participants throughout the follow-up, (2) the use of multi-informant and valid clinical assessments including gold standard diagnostic instruments, and (3) low dropout rates (<10% at 24 months). These strengths enable wane and us to determine whether the behavioural traits of ASD and related conditions may wax and to identify individuals who are at risk of such conditions as well as those whose symptoms may resolve over time. In addition, this cohort enables the investigation of determinants and outcomes of various behaviours displayed during infancy.

11.4 What We Found: HBC Study

The HBC Study team demonstrated that early neurodevelopmental trajectories of the five MSEL domains (gross motor, visual reception, fine motor, receptive language, and expressive language) by 24 months can be categorised into five classes using latent class growth analysis and using data from the HBC Study sample [67]. The effect of latent classes on distal outcome (i.e. a clinical diagnosis of ASD) has also been investigated [68]. Using a classical approach, individuals were assigned to the latent class based on posterior probabilities, following which the association between the observed outcome and the latent classes was examined by treating the class membership as a known variable. Feingold et al. [69] reported that using this classical approach underestimates the associations between latent class and outcome. To avoid such underestimation and obtain unbiased estimates, we utilised a one-step analysis, in which the outcome variable was included in the latent class model.

In the present study, we identified five trajectories as follows (Fig. 11.2). The high normal class (11.5%; n = 110) was characterised by relatively accelerated development in all five domains. The growth progress in the normal class (n = 468; 49.2%) was nearly linear and parallel along the mean value of 50 over the period of analysis. Infants in the low normal class (n = 202; 21.2%) exhibited a slight delay during the early developmental stages but matched the progress of infants in the normal and high normal classes by 24 months of age. These three classes were considered "normal" because the trajectories were in the range of the mean ± 1 SD. The delayed class (n = 134; 14.1%) exhibited a downward deviation in

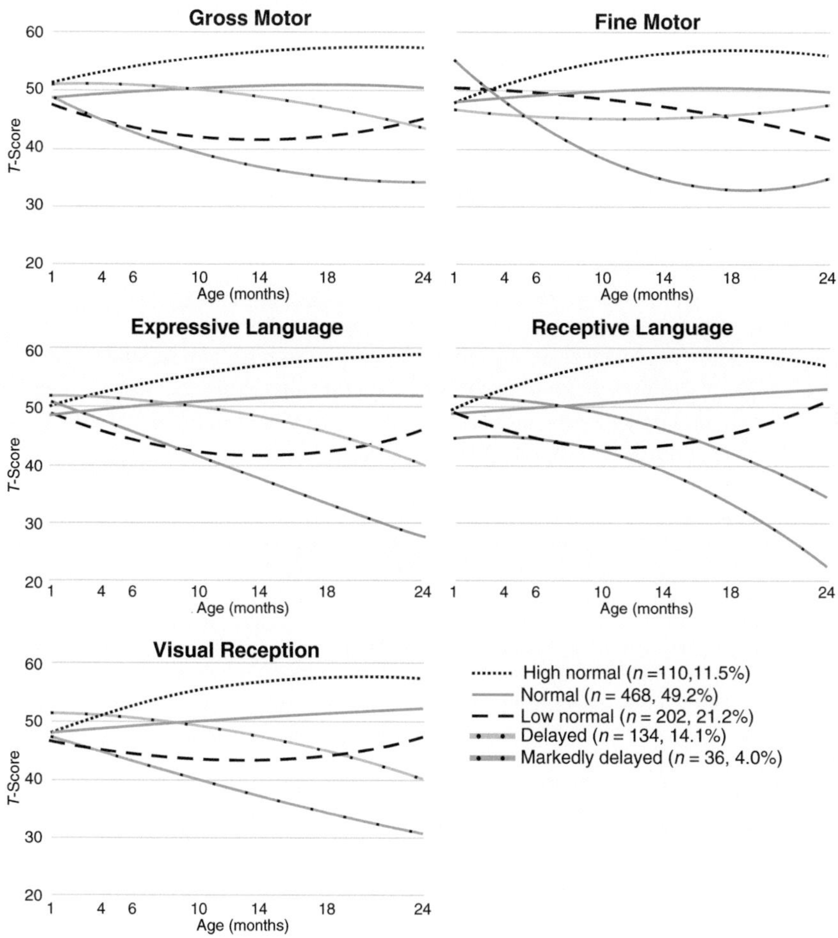

Fig. 11.2 The five trajectory classes of the Mullen Scales of Early Learning from 1 to 24 months of age

T-scores after around 12 months of age, particularly in the receptive language domain. The markedly delayed class ($n = 38$; 4.0%) was characterised by an overall delay from the early developmental stages, which was associated with marked delays in motor domains at an earlier stage and a somewhat later delay in language domains.

We further observed that the probability of ASD diagnosis was highest (32.6%) in the markedly delayed class. The probabilities of ASD diagnosis in the delayed and low normal classes were 6.4% and 4.0%, respectively. The probabilities of ASD diagnosis for the normal and high normal class were both 0%. Latent class odds ratios were not obtained because the probability of an ASD diagnosis for the reference class (normal) was 0%.

We also identified precedents for the two classes that show significant delay in the trajectories. The markedly delayed class was predicted by male sex (odds ratio 4.0; 95% CI 1.7–9.1), small for gestational age (2.8; 95% CI 1.0–7.5), and maternal education of shorter than 12 years (4.7; 95% CI 1.2–19.0). The delayed class was predicted by male sex (2.5; 95% CI 1.5–4.2), but also by preterm birth (4.4; 95% CI 1.6–12.6), and a 10-year increase in paternal age (1.9; 1.0–3.5).

11.5 Conclusion

Currently, the contribution of specific developmental trajectories to ASD risk remains unknown. However, in our general-population birth cohort study, approximately 40% of children belonging to three latent groups exhibited varying degrees of developmental delay by the age of 24 months. We observed an increased risk for ASD in these children. Further data are awaited.

Acknowledgements The authors thank Dr. Tetsuo Kato of the Kato Maternity Clinic for enrolling study participants. The authors are grateful to Drs. K. Sugihara, M. Sugimura, K. Takeuchi, K. Suzuki, Y. Murakami, Y. Koumura, Y. Miyabe, K. Hirai, Y. Nakamura, R. Koizumi, H. Murakami, Y. Kobayashi-Koumura, and K. Muramatsu-Kato and to all attending obstetricians for enrolling pregnant women to participate in the study. The authors thank the chief midwife, Ms. Kiyomi Hinoki, and all the midwives and staff at the Hamamatsu University School of Medicine maternity clinic, for enrolling participants.

Funding: This work is supported by Grants-in-Aid from the Ministry of Education, Culture, Sports, Science, and Technology of Japan (K.J. Tsuchiya, S. Takagai) and the SENSHIN Medical Research Foundation (K.J. Tsuchiya).

Conflict of Interest: None declared.

References

1. Bishop D, Rutter M. Neurodevelopmental disorders: conceptual issues. In: Rutter M, Bishop DVM, Pine DS, et al., editors. Rutter's child and adolescent psychiatry. 5th ed. Malden: Blackwell Publishing, Inc.; 2008. p. 32–41.

2. WHO. The ICD-10 classification of mental and behavioural disorders (ICD-10): the clinical descriptions and diagnostic guidelines. Geneva: World Health Organization; 1992.
3. American Psychiatric Assciation. Diagnostic and statistical manual. 5th ed. Washington DC: American Psychiatric Association; 2013.
4. Thomas R, Sanders S, Doust J, Beller E, Glasziou P. Prevalence of attention-deficit/hyperactivity disorder: a systematic review and meta-analysis. Pediatrics. 2015;135:e994–1001.
5. Rowland AS, Skipper BJ, Umbach DM, et al. The prevalence of ADHD in a population-based sample. J Atten Disord. 2015;19:741–54.
6. Rohde LA, Szobot C, Polanczyk G, Schmitz M, Martins S, Tramontina S. Attention-deficit/hyperactivity disorder in a diverse culture: do research and clinical findings support the notion of a cultural construct for the disorder? Biol Psychiatry. 2005;57:1436–41.
7. Polanczyk G, de Lima MS, Horta BL, Biederman J, Rohde LA. The worldwide prevalence of ADHD: a systematic review and metaregression analysis. Am J Psychiatry. 2007;164:942–8.
8. Erskine HE, Ferrari AJ, Nelson P, et al. Epidemiological modelling of attention-deficit/hyperactivity disorder and conduct disorder for the Global Burden of Disease Study 2010. J Child Psychol Psychiatry. 2013;54:1263–74.
9. Larson K, Russ SA, Kahn RS, Halfon N. Patterns of comorbidity, functioning, and service use for US children with ADHD, 2007. Pediatrics. 2011;127:462–70.
10. Agnew-Blais JC, Polanczyk GV, Danese A, Wertz J, Moffitt TE, Arseneault L. Evaluation of the persistence, remission, and emergence of attention-deficit/hyperactivity disorder in young adulthood. JAMA Psychiatry. 2016;73:713–20.
11. Van Naarden Braun K, Christensen D, Doernberg N, et al. Trends in the prevalence of autism spectrum disorder, cerebral palsy, hearing loss, intellectual disability, and vision impairment, metropolitan atlanta, 1991-2010. PLoS One. 2015;10:e0124120.
12. Centers for Disease Control and Prevention (CDC). Prevalence of autism spectrum disorder among children aged 8 years—autism and developmental disabilities monitoring network, 11 sites, United States, 2010. MMWR Surveill Summ. 2014;63:1–21.
13. Idring S, Lundberg M, Sturm H, et al. Changes in prevalence of autism spectrum disorders in 2001-2011: findings from the Stockholm youth cohort. J Autism Dev Disord. 2015;45:1766–73.
14. Elsabbagh M, Divan G, Koh YJ, et al. Global prevalence of autism and other pervasive developmental disorders. Autism Res. 2012;5:160–79.
15. Kim YS, Leventhal BL, Koh YJ, et al. Prevalence of autism spectrum disorders in a total population sample. Am J Psychiatry. 2011;168:904–12.
16. Howlin P. Outcomes in autism spectrum disorders. In: Volkmar FR, Paul R, Klin A, Cohen D, editors. Handbook of autism and pervasive developmental disorders. 3rd ed. Hoboken: Wiley; 2005. p. 201–20.
17. Wong C, Odom SL, Hume KA, et al. Evidence-based practices for children, youth, and young adults with autism spectrum disorder: a comprehensive review. J Autism Dev Disord. 2015;45(7):1951–66.
18. Taurines R, Schwenck C, Westerwald E, Sachse M, Siniatchkin M, Freitag C. ADHD and autism: differential diagnosis or overlapping traits? A selective review. Atten Defic Hyperact Disord. 2012;4:115–39.
19. Johnson MH, Gliga T, Jones E, Charman T. Annual research review: infant development, autism, and ADHD—early pathways to emerging disorders. J Child Psychol Psychiatry. 2015;56:228–47.
20. Franke N, Keown LJ, Sanders MR. An RCT of an online parenting program for parents of preschool-aged children with ADHD symptoms. J Atten Disord. 2016.; Sep 8. pii: 1087054716667598.
21. Pan PY, Yeh CB. Impact of depressive/anxiety symptoms on the quality of life of adolescents with ADHD: a community-based 1-year prospective follow-up study. Eur Child Adolesc Psychiatry. 2017;26(6):659–67.
22. Mazefsky CA, Folstein SE, Lainhart JE. Overrepresentation of mood and anxiety disorders in adults with autism and their first-degree relatives: what does it mean? Autism Res. 2008;1:193–7.

23. Mazefsky CA, Conner CM, Oswald DP. Association between depression and anxiety in high-functioning children with autism spectrum disorders and maternal mood symptoms. Autism Res. 2010;3:120–7.
24. Atladottir HO, Gyllenberg D, Langridge A, et al. The increasing prevalence of reported diagnoses of childhood psychiatric disorders: a descriptive multinational comparison. Eur Child Adolesc Psychiatry. 2015;24:173–83.
25. Sun X, Allison C, Matthews FE, et al. Prevalence of autism in mainland China, Hong Kong and Taiwan: a systematic review and meta-analysis. Mol Autism. 2013;4:7.
26. Wing L, Yeates SR, Brierley LM, Gould J. The prevalence of early childhood autism: comparison of administrative and epidemiological studies. Psychol Med. 1976;6:89–100.
27. Schechter R, Grether JK. Continuing increases in autism reported to California's developmental services system: mercury in retrograde. Arch Gen Psychiatry. 2008;65:19–24.
28. Parner ET, Schendel DE, Thorsen P. Autism prevalence trends over time in Denmark: changes in prevalence and age at diagnosis. Arch Pediatr Adolesc Med. 2008;162:1150–6.
29. Baxter AJ, Brugha TS, Erskine HE, Scheurer RW, Vos T, Scott JG. The epidemiology and global burden of autism spectrum disorders. Psychol Med. 2015;45:601–13.
30. Horlin C, Falkmer M, Parsons R, Albrecht MA, Falkmer T. The cost of autism spectrum disorders. PLoS One. 2014;9:e106552.
31. Lavelle TA, Weinstein MC, Newhouse JP, Munir K, Kuhlthau KA, Prosser LA. Economic burden of childhood autism spectrum disorders. Pediatrics. 2014;133:e520–9.
32. Cadman T, Eklund H, Howley D, et al. Caregiver burden as people with autism spectrum disorder and attention-deficit/hyperactivity disorder transition into adolescence and adulthood in the United Kingdom. J Am Acad Child Adolesc Psychiatry. 2012;51:879–88.
33. Vohra R, Madhavan S, Sambamoorthi U, St Peter C. Access to services, quality of care, and family impact for children with autism, other developmental disabilities, and other mental health conditions. Autism. 2014;18:815–26.
34. Ozonoff S, Young GS, Steinfeld MB, et al. How early do parent concerns predict later autism diagnosis? J Dev Behav Pediatr. 2009;30:367–75.
35. Zwaigenbaum L, Bryson S, Rogers T, Roberts W, Brian J, Szatmari P. Behavioral manifestations of autism in the first year of life. Int J Dev Neurosci. 2005;23:143–52.
36. Zwaigenbaum L, Bryson S, Garon N. Early identification of autism spectrum disorders. Behav Brain Res. 2013;251:133–46.
37. Fein D, Barton M, Eigsti IM, et al. Optimal outcome in individuals with a history of autism. J Child Psychol Psychiatry. 2013;54:195–205.
38. Helt M, Kelley E, Kinsbourne M, et al. Can children with autism recover? If so, how? Neuropsychol Rev. 2008;18:339–66.
39. Landa R, Garrett-Mayer E. Development in infants with autism spectrum disorders: a prospective study. J Child Psychol Psychiatry. 2006;47:629–38.
40. Szatmari P, Georgiades S, Duku E, et al. Developmental trajectories of symptom severity and adaptive functioning in an inception cohort of preschool children with autism spectrum disorder. JAMA Psychiatry. 2015;72:276–83.
41. Luyster RJ, Seery A, Talbott MR, Tager-Flusberg H. Identifying early-risk markers and developmental trajectories for language impairment in neurodevelopmental disorders. Dev Disabil Res Rev. 2011;17:151–9.
42. Landa RJ, Gross AL, Stuart EA, Faherty A. Developmental trajectories in children with and without autism spectrum disorders: the first 3 years. Child Dev. 2013;84:429–42.
43. Vorstman JA, Parr JR, Moreno-De-Luca D, Anney RJ, Nurnberger JI Jr, Hallmayer JF. Autism genetics: opportunities and challenges for clinical translation. Nat Rev Genet. 2017;18(6):362–76.
44. Banaschewski T, Becker K, Scherag S, Franke B, Coghill D. Molecular genetics of attention-deficit/hyperactivity disorder: an overview. Eur Child Adolesc Psychiatry. 2010;19:237–57.
45. Franke B, Neale BM, Faraone SV. Genome-wide association studies in ADHD. Hum Genet. 2009;126:13–50.
46. Bohnert KM, Breslau N. Stability of psychiatric outcomes of low birth weight: a longitudinal investigation. Arch Gen Psychiatry. 2008;65:1080–6.

47. Breslau N, Brown GG, DelDotto JE, et al. Psychiatric sequelae of low birth weight at 6 years of age. J Abnorm Child Psychol. 1996;24:385–400.
48. Lampi KM, Lehtonen L, Tran PL, et al. Risk of autism spectrum disorders in low birth weight and small for gestational age infants. J Pediatr. 2012;161:830–6.
49. Kolevzon A, Gross R, Reichenberg A. Prenatal and perinatal risk factors for autism: a review and integration of findings. Arch Pediatr Adolesc Med. 2007;161:326–33.
50. Hvolgaard Mikkelsen S, Olsen J, Bech BH, Obel C. Parental age and attention-deficit/hyperactivity disorder (ADHD). Int J Epidemiol. 2017;46(2):409–20.
51. Tsuchiya KJ, Matsumoto K, Yagi A, et al. Reliability and validity of autism diagnostic interview-revised, Japanese version. J Autism Dev Disord. 2013;43:643–62.
52. Hultman CM, Sandin S, Levine SZ, Lichtenstein P, Reichenberg A. Advancing paternal age and risk of autism: new evidence from a population-based study and a meta-analysis of epidemiological studies. Mol Psychiatry. 2011;16:1203–12.
53. Ode A, Kallen K, Gustafsson P, et al. Fetal exposure to perfluorinated compounds and attention deficit hyperactivity disorder in childhood. PLoS One. 2014;9:e95891.
54. Liew Z, Ritz B, von Ehrenstein OS, et al. Attention deficit/hyperactivity disorder and childhood autism in association with prenatal exposure to perfluoroalkyl substances: a nested case-control study in the Danish National Birth Cohort. Environ Health Perspect. 2015;123:367–73.
55. Volk HE, Lurmann F, Penfold B, Hertz-Picciotto I, McConnell R. Traffic-related air pollution, particulate matter, and autism. JAMA Psychiatry. 2013;70:71–7.
56. Volk HE, Hertz-Picciotto I, Delwiche L, Lurmann F, McConnell R. Residential proximity to freeways and autism in the CHARGE study. Environ Health Perspect. 2011;119:873–7.
57. Yoshida K, Yamashita H, Ueda M, Tashiro N. Postnatal depression in Japanese mothers and the reconsideration of 'Satogaeri bunben'. Pediatr Int. 2001;43:189–93.
58. First MB, Spitzer RL, Gibbon M, Williams JBW. Structured clinical interview for DSM-IV axis I disorders (version 2.0). Arlington: American Psychiatric Publishing, Inc.; 1996.
59. Mullen EM. Mullen scales of early learning: AGS Edition. Minneapolis: Pearson Assessments; 1995.
60. Wechsler D. Manual for the Wechsler preschool and primary scale of intelligence. San Antonio: The Psychological Corporation; 1967.
61. Wechsler D, Golombok S, Rust J. Wechsler intelligence scale for children—Third Edition UK (WISC-IIIUK). London: The Psychological Corporation; 1992.
62. Robins DL, Fein D, Barton ML, Green JA. The Modified Checklist for Autism in Toddlers: an initial study investigating the early detection of autism and pervasive developmental disorders. J Autism Dev Disord. 2001;31:131–44.
63. Kamio Y, Inada N. A preliminary study on the early detection of pervasive developmental disorders at 18-month check-up. Seishin Igaku. 2006;48:981–90.
64. Lord C, Risi S, Lambrecht L, et al. The autism diagnostic observation schedule-generic: a standard measure of social and communication deficits associated with the spectrum of autism. J Autism Dev Disord. 2000;30:205–23.
65. Filipek PA, Accardo PJ, Ashwal S, et al. Practice parameter: screening and diagnosis of autism: report of the Quality Standards Subcommittee of the American Academy of Neurology and the Child Neurology Society. Neurology. 2000;55:468–79.
66. DuPaul GJ, Power TJ, McGoey K, Ikeda M, Anastopoulos AD. Reliability and validity of parent and teacher ratings of attention-deficit/hyperactivity disorder symptoms. J Psychoeduc Assess. 1998;16:55–8.
67. Nishimura T, Takei N, Tsuchiya KJ, Asano R, Mori N. Identification of neurodevelopmental trajectories in infancy and of risk factors affecting deviant development: a longitudinal birth cohort study. Int J Epidemiol. 2016;45:543–53.
68. Nishimura T, Takei N, Tsuchiya KJ. Neurodevelopmental trajectory during infancy and diagnosis of autism spectrum disorder as an outcome at 32 months of age. Epidemiology (in press).
69. Feingold A, Tiberio SS, Capaldi DM. New approaches for examining associations with latent categorical variables: applications to substance abuse and aggression. Psychol Addict Behav. 2014;28:257–67.

Chapter 12
Birth Cohort Consortium of Asia (BiCCA): Current Children's Environmental Health Issues in Asia and Future Perspectives

Mei-Huei Chen, Sharon Ng, Meng-Shan Tsai, Ching-Chun Lin, and Pau-Chung Chen

Abstract Background: The environment is an important factor which not only may influence children's health at early life but also may lead to adverse consequences on later health. However, children in Asia are facing both traditional environmental hazards and new pediatric morbidities. A collaboration platform of Asian birth cohort studies to promote children's environmental health is warranted.

Methods: The Birth Cohort Consortium of Asia (BiCCA) was co-established in 2011 by the principal investigators of three birth cohorts in Asia including the Taiwan Birth Panel Study (TBPS), the Mothers and Children's Environmental

M.-H. Chen
Institute of Population Health Sciences, National Health Research Institutes, Miaoli, Taiwan

Department of Pediatrics, National Taiwan University Hospital Yun-Lin Branch, Yunlin, Taiwan

Department of Pediatrics, National Taiwan University College of Medicine and Hospital, Taipei, Taiwan

S. Ng
Department of Obstetrics and Gynaecology, Yong Loo Lin School of Medicine, National University of Singapore, National University Health System, Singapore, Singapore

M.-S. Tsai · C.-C. Lin
Institute of Occupational Medicine and Industrial Hygiene, National Taiwan University College of Public Health, Taipei, Taiwan

P.-C. Chen (✉)
Institute of Occupational Medicine and Industrial Hygiene, National Taiwan University College of Public Health, Taipei, Taiwan

Department of Environmental and Occupational Medicine, National Taiwan University Hospital and National Taiwan University College of Medicine, Taipei, Taiwan

Department of Public Health, National Taiwan University College of Public Health, Taipei, Taiwan
e-mail: pchen@ntu.edu.tw

F. Sata et al. (eds.), *Pre-emptive Medicine: Public Health Aspects of Developmental Origins of Health and Disease*, Current Topics in Environmental Health and Preventive Medicine, https://doi.org/10.1007/978-981-13-2194-8_12

Health Study (MOCEH), and the Hokkaido Study on Environment and Children's Health (Hokkaido Study). The related informations of environmental exposure and health outcome from participating cohorts have been published.

Results: Up to date (October, 2017), BiCCA includes 27 birth cohorts with approximately 80,000 study subjects that were conducted in 13 Asian countries. The geographical distribution of the cohort studies is uneven and assessment tools are diverse. Certain environmental neurotoxins have been identified; however, the exploration to critical environmental issues is not comprehensive. Targeted research collaboration is warranted and still ongoing.

Conclusions: The BiCCA provides an information exchange platform for birth cohort in Asian countries. Multidisciplinary collaboration and state-of-the-art technology application should initiate to identify specific regional environmental threats and improve the health of children in Asia.

Keywords Birth cohorts · Asia · Child environmental health

Abbreviations

BCSM	Birth Cohort Study in Mongolia—Towards Solving Global Problems in the Maternal and Child Health
BiCCA	Birth Cohort Consortium of Asia
BienHoa study	BienHoa Dioxin Cohort study
CHECK	Children's Health and Environmental Chemicals in Korea
CLHNS	Cebu Longitudinal Health and Nutritional Survey
COCOA	Cohort for Childhood Origin of Asthma and Allergic Diseases
DaDoCiV	Dioxin and Development of Children in Vietnam
DaNang study	DaNang Dioxin Cohort study
DOHaD	Developmental Origins of Health and Disease
EDC study	Environment and Development of Children Study
GUSTO	Growing up in Singapore Towards Healthy Outcomes
HBC study	Hamamatsu Birth Cohort for Mothers and Children
Hokkaido study	Hokkaido cohort: Hokkaido Study on Environment and Children's Health
HRBC	Harvard Reproductive and Birth Cohort
KCHS	Kalutara Children's Health Study
LWBC	Laizhou Wan Birth Cohort
MISC	Mother-Infant Study Cohort
MOCEH	Mothers and Children's Environmental Health Study
Nepali	Nepali Birth Cohort Study in Chitwan Valley
NJMUBC	Nanjing Medical University Birth Cohort
PCBs	Polychlorinated biphenyls
PFASs	Perfluoroalkyl substances
PSKC	Panel Study on Korean Children

Sapporo study	Sapporo cohort: Hokkaido Study on Environment and Children's Health
SBC	Shanghai Birth Cohort
TBPS	Taiwan Birth Panel Study
TEC	Taiwan Early-Life Cohort
TMICS	Taiwan Maternal and Infant Cohort Study
TSCD	The Tohoku Study of Child Development
UGAAR	Ulaanbaatar Gestation and Air Pollution Research
USM Pregnancy Cohort Study	Universiti Sains Malaysia Pregnancy Cohort Study

12.1 Introduction

The World Health Organization (WHO) had reported that 23% of global deaths and 26% of deaths among children under 5 are due to modifiable environmental factors [1]. Children's environmental health issues may vary widely with regional development but may also be affected by globalization simultaneously. Asia contains more than half of children population in the world. The general environmental factors such as climate, geography, ethnic, and cultures diverse greatly. Moreover, poor, wealthy, underdeveloped, or rapid industrialization countries are all included in this area. Coexistence of traditional environment hazards and new emerging threats is a complex challenge. These phenomena highlight the uniqueness and importance of children's environmental health in Asia [2, 3].

12.2 Child's Environmental Health Burden

The burden of environmental-related disease is unevenly distributed, with greatest exposure to children in developing or low-income countries. Although the primary health issues of children in developing countries are low birth weight, malnutrition, and infectious diseases, they are also facing new pediatric morbidity including allergic diseases, neurobehavioral problems, and overweight and obesity same as children in developed countries [4, 5]. On the other aspect, traditional environmental hazards such as unsafe water, contaminated food, and myriad of toxic chemicals are major threats to children in developing countries, while environmental tobacco smoke, air pollution, and food-related persistent and nonpersistent endocrine-disruptive chemical exposure attract more attention in developed countries. Nevertheless, the aforementioned boundaries (or classifications) have been broken due to the relocation of heavy and traditional industries into developing countries and frequent international exchanges. The circulation of dust, air, water, and food chain all facilitate the ubiquitous distribution of air pollutants, persistent organic pollutants, or contaminants of emerging concern that originate from industrialization. Therefore, children's environmental health is both of regional and global importance.

12.3 Role of Birth Cohort Studies

The foundation to promote environmental child health in Asia is to recognize the major environmental threats in each specific region or country, figure out their temporal trends, and establish the scientific evidences for their health hazards. Birth cohort is an ideal design to investigate health outcomes following environmental exposure during critical developmental period. In Asia, some birth cohort studies have lasted for years and contributed to important scientific issues such as environmental tobacco smoke. Until recently, the necessity of nationwide or large-scale birth cohorts has been emphasized as well. It's the optimal timing to establish a collaboration platform for Asian birth cohorts. Information derived from preexisting studies may be harmonized by redefined standardized exposure and outcome variables. Integration should increase statistical power through an enlarged set of data, allowing the researcher to examine rare events or strengthen the scientific evidence of causality. The pathogenesis of environmental toxicants could be further explored via comparisons between diverse exposure levels and genetic variation derived from different studies. The unsolved issues and priority could be identified. The updated or consensus of methodology for exposure and outcome assessments may further provide foundation for next-generation or nationwide birth cohorts. The ultimate goal is to translate scientific knowledge derived from multiple studies or countries to policy-making or strategy implementation to promote environmental health of children in Asia and beyond.

12.4 Birth Cohort Consortium of Asia (BiCCA)

The Birth Cohort Consortium of Asia (BiCCA) was co-established in 2011 by the principal investigators (PIs) of the following three birth cohorts in Asia: the Taiwan Birth Panel Study (TBPS) from Taiwan (PI: Chen), the Mothers and Children's Environmental Health Study (MOCEH) from Korea (PI: Ha), and the Hokkaido Study on Environment and Children's Health (Hokkaido Study) from Japan (PI: Kishi). The aims are to facilitate the exchange of knowledge and collaboration between cohorts and researchers and to explore the future needs of children in Asia. Several symposia/seminar, workshop, and PI meetings were held to build capacity related to inclusion criteria, inventory, profile paper, and organization bylaws.

Up to date (October, 2017), BiCCA includes 27 birth cohorts with approximately 80,000 study subjects that were conducted in 13 Asian countries (Fig. 12.1), including China (3 cohorts), Japan (4), Malaysia (1), Mongolia (2), the Philippines (1), the Republic of Korea (5), Singapore (1), Taiwan (3), and Vietnam (3) in

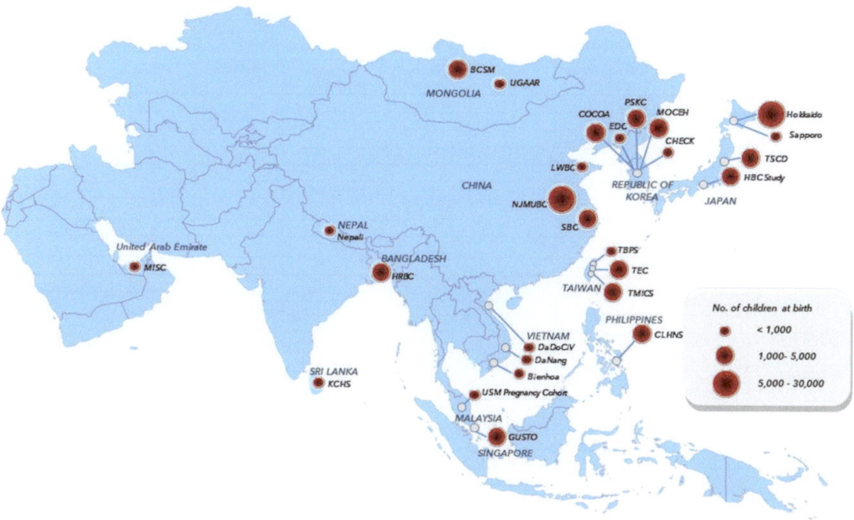

Fig. 12.1 Asian birth cohort studies collaborating in BiCCA. Adapted from Kishi R. et al. Birth cohort consortium of Asia: current and future perspectives. Epidemiology 2017

Western Pacific Region; Bangladesh (1), Nepal (1), and Sri Lanka (1) in the Southeast Asia Region; and the United Arab Emirates (1) in the Eastern Mediterranean Region. The enrolment period and numbers of participants of each cohort varied widely. The oldest cohort, CLHNS (Cebu Longitudinal Health and Nutritional Survey), was established in 1983, while the newest one, MISC (Mother-Infant Study Cohort), was started since 2015. Most of the cohorts recruited mothers during pregnancy or at birth. The only two preconception cohorts were NJMUBC (Nanjing Medical University Birth Cohort) and SBC (Shanghai Birth Cohort) from China, and biosamples from biological father were collected. COCOA (Cohort for Childhood Origin of Asthma and Allergic Diseases) also collected blood and DNA of the biological father. Cohorts in Malaysia, Nepal, and Vietnam recruited only 100–200 participants; NJMUBC established since 2014 planned to enroll 30,000 mother-infant pairs [6]. While most of the cohort studies in BiCCA focused on environmental pollutants, BCSM (Birth Cohort Study in Mongolia—Towards Solving Global Problems in the Maternal and Child Health), CLHNS, GUSTO (Growing up in Singapore Towards Health Outcomes), MISC, Nepali (Nepali Birth Cohort Study in Chitwan Valley), and USM Pregnancy Cohort Study (Universiti Sains Malaysia Pregnancy Cohort Study) were designed to investigate the role of nutrients. Those cohorts were marked as gray column in Table 12.1. GUSTO even performed comprehensive measurements of body composition of children including skinfolds and magnetic resonance imaging.

Table 2.1 Measurements of selected environmental exposure and nutrients intake of participating studies in Birth Cohort Consortium of Aisa

Nation	Cohort Name	Outdoor air pollutions	Tobacco smoke[a]	Heavy metals[b]	Diet and nutrition[c]	Pesticides	POPs	non-POPs EDC
BANGLADESH	HRBC			Arsenic				
CHINA	LWBC			v	v	v	v	v
	NJMUBC	v	v	v	v	v	v	v
	SBC			v	v	v	v	v
JAPAN	HBC Study				v			
	Hokkaido		v		Folate only		v	v
	Sapporo		v	Mercury	v	v	v	v
	TSCD			v	v	v	v	
KOREA	CHECK			v	v	v	v	v
	COCOA	v	v		v			v
	EDC study	v	v	v	v		v	v
	MOCEH	v	v	v	v			v
	PSKC		v					
MALAYSIA	USM Pregnancy Cohort		v		v			
MONGOLIA	BCSM				Fish intake only			
	UGAAR	v						
NEPAL	Nepali			v	v			
PHILIPPINES	CLHNS				v			
SINGAPORE	GUSTO	v	v		v			
SRI LANKA	KCHS	v						
TAIWAN	TBPS		v	v	v	v	v	v
	TEC	v		v	v		v	
	TMICS		v	v	v	v	v	v
VIETNAM	BienHoa study						dioxin	
	DaDoCiV						dioxin	
	DaNang study						dioxin	
UNITED ARAB EMIRATE	MISC				Infant feeding practices			

Those cohorts designed to investigate the role of nutrients were marked with a gray column

[a]Biomarker measurement available

[b]Metals such as aluminum, antimony, arsenic, barium, beryllium, cadmium, cesium, chromium, cobalt, gallium, lead, mercury, molybdenum, nickel, platinum, thallium, thorium, tungsten, and uranium are included

[c]Essential elements such as manganese, zinc, copper, selenium, and iron

12.5 Brief Summary of Cohort Characteristics

Table 12.1 shows the selected environmental exposure of participating studies in BiCCA. Certain cohorts target their studies on specific environment pollutants, for example, Harvard Reproductive and Birth Cohort (HRBC) in Bangladesh investigated the impact of arsenic exposure, Ulaanbaatar Gestation and Air Pollution Research (UGAAR) Study in Mongolia explored the health effects of air pollution, the Kalutara Children's Health Study (KCHS) in Sri Lanka focused mainly on exposure to PM2.5 and black carbon, and three small cohorts in Vietnam focused on toxicity of dioxin. Cohorts in Japan, Korea, and Taiwan concern not only on traditional environmental hazards such as heavy metals and/or pesticides but also on persistent organic pollutants or other endocrine disrupters. Exceptions are Hamamatsu Birth Cohort for Mothers and Children (HBC) study in Japan which investigated the trajectories of children neurodevelopment and the Panel Study on Korean Children (PSKC) which aims to collect data on the characteristics of children's growth and development. Cohorts in China, one of the fastest growing economies, were established within the recent 5 years and do consider a variety of environmental pollutants. As expected, tobacco smoke is a universal concern regardless of status of industrialization or urbanization. Although only one third of cohorts record outdoor air pollution, the health hazards of these transboundary pollutants need special attention.

12.6 Knowledge Derived from BiCCA

Bicca provide the very first step to integrate the public information related to birth cohorts in Aisa on public. With this platform, we found that the geographical distribution of the cohort studies is uneven and exploration to critical environmental issues is not comprehensive. The experiences of developed countries to deal with traditional pollutants are worth sharing such as removal of lead from gasoline, the mercury pollution reduction project, and antismoking campaigns [2]. Meanwhile, contaminants of emerging concern, outdoor air pollution, or climate change could be the future common enemy for children in Asia. Despite the main health issues focusing on fetal growth, pregnancy outcome, growth and obesity, allergic disease and immune function, neurodevelopmental and behavioral problems, and endocrine function, the diverse assessment tools for neurobehavioral status could be the largest challenge. A recent review summarized relevant epidemiologic evidence for cohorts in Asia and points out the potential neurotoxicity of mercury, environmental tobacco smoke, polychlorinated biphenyls (PCBs), and perfluoroalkyl substances (PFASs) on children [7]. The initiation of targeted research collaboration within BiCCA and data harmonization has started. The BiCCA still welcomes birth cohorts in Asia to join us. Enquiries and initial approaches regarding membership or detailed information are welcome (http://www.bicca.org/).

12.7 Future Perspective Through Collaboration

Traditionally, the paradigm of Developmental Origins of Health and Disease (DOHaD) has focused on influences of nutrition status during early life on health across the lifespan. Environmental child health research have specifically investigated exposure to unfavorable chemicals from environmental or occupational setting during prenatal and/or early postnatal period and its impact on the occurrence of diseases later. Nevertheless, co-exposure and interactions between nutrient elements, environmental toxicants, and genetic variation are a reality in the living environment. For instance, predator fish consumption provides a variety of essential nutrients such as polyunsaturated fatty acid and selenium but also has been recognized as one of the major sources of persistent organic pollutants including methylmercury, PFASs, dioxin, and dioxin-like compounds in the general population [8]. Combined data from Taiwanese and Korean birth cohorts showed that fish consumption and cord blood mercury level influenced birth weight at opposite direction by path analysis [9]. In addition, early life events especially during the critical fetal development period predispose not only to childhood illness but also to increased risk of adulthood morbidity and mortality. Accumulating evidences have supported that maternal medical conditions (e.g., preeclampsia, gestation diabetes mellitus, anemia, etc.), malnutrition, in utero exposure to environmental tobacco smoke, heavy metals, and endocrine-disruptive chemicals may affect fetal growth [10, 11] and may be associated with increased risk of low birth weight [12] and non-communicable diseases in adulthood. The concept of exposome, which refers to measures that reflect all exposure events of an individual during a lifetime and how those exposures relate to disease, provides new insight to cope with the health research related to the beneficial effect of nutrients and toxic effect of environmental pollutants [13]. Along with the advancement of "omic" technologies, the exploration of biological functions such as DNA methylation or microbiome pattern that are influenced by maternal or fetal exposome becomes feasible and should contribute to the understanding of causal relationship between exposure and health.

12.8 Challenge of Child's Environmental Health Research

Prevention is the core concept of children's environmental health. However, low-dose multipollutant exposure in human daily life is unavoidable; even the regulation of toxic chemicals or workplace safety control decreases the incidence of severe intoxication or high-dose environmental contamination. In regard to health hazard, the effect for single pollutant exposure may be small, but the impact of mixture exposure is usually unknown and lacks scientific evidence. Furthermore, the differences of individual susceptibility and gene-environment interaction are challenges for clinical assessment of environmental threats. Unlike a specific causal-relationship as infectious pathogen and disease, the role of environmental pollutans on the occurence of disease could be only one of the causative or trigger factors. Co-existance with other adverse factors such as life style are needed to affect health. The exposure factor for risk assessment varies by physiological and behavioral differences among different age groups [14]. These uncertainties may underestimate the health effects of environmental pollutants, especially for vulnerable pregnant women and children. Ultimately, how to apply the state-of-the-art technique in analysis and risk assessment in preventing children's environmental threats is the key of knowledge translation to implementation.

12.9 Conclusions

The establishment of BiCCA provides a platform for information exchange related to basic characteristics, environmental exposure measurements, and outcome assessment of birth cohorts in Asia. Therefore, a multidisciplinary collaboration with different professionals has to be initiated, not only the integration of preexisting knowledge but also the application of state-of-art technologies to maximize the advantage of the birth cohort research design. Ultimately, these efforts should contribute to improving children's environmental health.

Acknowledgments This manuscript was supported by grants from the Ministry of Science and Technology (MOST-105-2314-B-002-048-MY2), Taiwan, and the Environmental Medicine Collaboration Center (NTUH-103-A123, NTUH-104-A123, and NTUH-105-A123), National Taiwan University Hospital.

References

1. Prüss-Üstün A, Wolf J, Corvalán CF, Bos R, Neira MP. Preventing disease through healthy environments: a global assessment of the burden of disease from environmental risks. World Health Organization; 2016. http://www.who.int/iris/handle/10665/204585.
2. Suk WA, Ruchirawat KM, Balakrishnan K, et al. Environmental threats to children's health in Southeast Asia and the Western Pacific. Environ Health Perspect. 2003;111:1340–7.
3. World Health Organization. Children's environmental health-annual report 2009. http://www.who.int/ceh/publications/en/. Accessed 29 Oct 2017.
4. Landrigan PJ, Etzel RA. Text book of children's environmental health. Oxford: Oxford University Press; 2014.
5. American Academy of Pediatrics Council on Environmental Health. In: Etzel RA, editor. Pediatric environmental health. 3rd ed. Elk Grove Village: American Academy of Pediatrics; 2012.
6. Kishi R, Zhang JJ, Ha EH, Chen PC, et al. Birth cohort consortium of Asia: current and future perspectives. Epidemiology. 2017;28(Suppl 1):S19–34.
7. Tsai MS, Chen MH, Lin CC, et al. Children's environmental health based on birth cohort studies in Asia. Sci Total Environ. 2017;609:396–409.
8. Kishi R, Nakajima T, Goudarzi H, et al. The Association of prenatal exposure to perfluorinated chemicals with maternal essential and long-chain polyunsaturated fatty acids during pregnancy and the birth weight of their offspring: the Hokkaido Study. Environ Health Perspect. 2015;123:1038–45.
9. Kim BM, Chen MH, Chen PC, et al. Path analysis of prenatal mercury levels and birth weights in Korean and Taiwanese birth cohorts. Sci Total Environ. 2017;605–606:1003–10.
10. Snijder CA, Heederik D, Pierik FH, et al. Fetal growth and prenatal exposure to bisphenol A: the generation R study. Environ Health Perspect. 2013;121:393–8.
11. Wang N, Cheng J, Han B, et al. Exposure to severe famine in the prenatal or postnatal period and the development of diabetes in adulthood: an observational study. Diabetologia. 2017;60:262–9.
12. Birks L, Casas M, Garcia AM, et al. Occupational exposure to endocrine-disrupting chemicals and birth weight and length of gestation: a European meta-analysis. Environ Health Perspect. 2016;124:1785–93.
13. Wild CP. The exposome: from concept to utility. Int J Epidemiol. 2012;41:24–32.
14. United States Environmental Protection Agency. Child-specific exposure factors handbook (2008, Final report). https://cfpub.epa.gov/ncea/risk/recordisplay.cfm?deid=199243. Accessed 29 Oct 2017.

Appendix A

Southampton Women's Survey (SWS)

Cyrus Cooper

<table>
<tr><td>Name</td><td colspan="3">Southampton Women's Survey</td><td colspan="2">Abbreviation</td><td>SWS</td></tr>
<tr><td>Homepage</td><td colspan="6">www.swsurvey.soton.ac.uk or www.mrc.soton.ac.uk/sws/</td></tr>
<tr><td rowspan="2">Recruited number</td><td>Children</td><td>3158</td><td>Mothers</td><td>12,583</td><td>Fathers</td><td>3158</td></tr>
<tr><td>Brothers/sisters</td><td></td><td>Grandparents</td><td></td><td>Others</td><td></td></tr>
<tr><td>Date of enrollment</td><td>Start</td><td colspan="2">1998</td><td>End</td><td colspan="2">2002</td></tr>
<tr><td>Principal investigator(s)</td><td colspan="3">Professor Hazel Inskip
Professor Cyrus Cooper</td><td>E-mail</td><td colspan="2">hmi@mrc.soton.ac.uk
cc@mrc.soton.ac.uk</td></tr>
<tr><td>Contact person(s)</td><td colspan="3">Professor Cyrus Cooper</td><td>E-mail</td><td colspan="2">cc@mrc.soton.ac.uk</td></tr>
<tr><td>Aims</td><td colspan="6">The Southampton Women's Survey was established to assess the influence of factors operating before conception and during pregnancy on the health and development of the offspring. Non-pregnant young women were recruited, and their subsequent offspring are being followed up. Few other longitudinal studies of children have data on the tempo of prenatal growth, and none in high-income countries have information recorded before pregnancy</td></tr>
</table>

(continued)

F. Sata et al. (eds.), *Pre-emptive Medicine: Public Health Aspects of Developmental Origins of Health and Disease*, Current Topics in Environmental Health and Preventive Medicine, https://doi.org/10.1007/978-981-13-2194-8

Public health activities	The Southampton Women's Survey has a dedicated website covering information for the public, for study members, and for researchers. Newsletters are sent to participants at appropriate intervals Child participants in the SWS are strongly represented on the local hospital's Public and Patient Involvement Adolescent Panel, which is consulted about future SWS follow-up waves Results from the SWS have led to the development of interventions studies aimed at improving public health. Notable interventions include vitamin D supplementation in pregnant women to improve their children's bone health (MAVIDOS), a combined probiotic and nutritional supplement before and during pregnancy to improve maternal glucose tolerance around 28 weeks' gestation (NiPPeR), a combined vitamin D with health behaviour change ("Healthy Conversation Skills") intervention to improve diet and body composition in the mothers and children (SPRING) and an educational intervention in teenagers (LifeLab) SWS findings have contributed to public health policy in Southampton and the local area (with contributions from the SWS team featuring in the Public Health Annual Report from time to time) as well as informing national and international guidance for women in pregnancy and those planning to conceive
Key reference	Inskip HM, Godfrey KM, Robinson SM, Law CM, Barker DJ, Cooper C. Cohort profile: The Southampton Women's Survey. Int J Epidemiol. 2006;90:42–8.

Western Australian Pregnancy Cohort (Raine) Study

Peter Eastwood

Name	Western Australian Pregnancy Cohort (Raine) Study			**Abbreviation**		Raine Study
Homepage	http://www.rainestudy.org.au/					
Recruited number	**Children**	2868	**Mothers**	2900	**Fathers**	2900
	Brothers/sisters		**Grandparents**		**Others**	
Date of enrollment	**Start**	1989		**End**	ongoing	
Principal investigator(s)	Professor Peter Eastwood, Professor Leon Straker			**E-mail**	Peter.Eastwood@health.wa.gov.au L.Straker@curtin.edu.au	
Contact person(s)	Professor Peter Eastwood			**E-mail**	Peter.Eastwood@health.wa.gov.au	
Aims	The Raine Study is one of the largest successful prospective cohorts of pregnancy, childhood, adolescence and now young adulthood to be carried out anywhere in the world. Initiated in 1989, the aim was to utilise intrauterine, perinatal and childhood data including lifestyle behaviours and environmental exposures to ascertain the relative contributions of familial risk factors, fetal growth, placental development and environmental insults to health precursors and outcomes. The purpose of the Raine Study now is to improve human health and well-being by studying the life course of a cohort of Western Australians from before birth onwards					

(continued)

Public health activities	Prospective longitudinal data has now been collected by questionnaire, clinical assessment and biological sample analysis at multiple time points through pregnancy, infancy, childhood, adolescence and young adulthood—specifically at 18 and 36 weeks gestation, birth and 1, 2, 3, 5, 8, 10, 14, 17, 20 and 22 years of age In addition to bringing the index participants (Generation 2), follow-up of the cohort parents (Generation 1) is conducted. A follow-up of the cohort offspring children (Generation 3) of the index participants is underway. Major challenges include retention of cohort participants, procuring funding to maintain the cohort and collect new data, enhancing infrastructure support to cope with increased data and activity and translation of discoveries into policy and practice **Public Health Research Activity** The Raine Study is a rich resource for researchers investigating the developmental origins of health and disease. The Raine Study has contributed to over two decades of scientific discovery with over 400 publications in peer-reviewed scientific journals. Examples of public health research utilising the rich data available in the Raine Study include the following. Genetic variations have been identified using genome-wide association studies which are associated with obesity [1] and asthma [2]. Life stressors for the mother during pregnancy have been associated with blood pressure in the offspring as young adults [3]. Smoking by the mother during pregnancy has been associated with asthma in the offspring as adolescents [4]. Gestational hypertension has been associated with poor mental health trajectories across childhood [5]. Exposure to phthalates during pregnancy has been related to reduced ovarian reserve in offspring in adolescence [6] The Raine Study has an established consumer representative group who provide an important consultative and collaborative role on research proposals and cohort management issues. The group has input into the content of all communication with study members and is consulted on areas for future research. The Raine Study produces newsletters, information booklets, cards and health information and provides individual results back to participants. Events are organised to commemorate significant events (e.g. kst birthday). The Raine Study has a website accessible to participants, researchers and the public (www.rainestudy.org.au) 1. Bradfield JP, Taal HR, Timpson NJ, Scherag A, Lecoeur C, Warrington NM, et al. A genome-wide association meta-analysis identifies new childhood obesity loci. Nat Genet. 2012;44(5):526–31. 2. Ferreira MA, Matheson MC, Duffy DL, Marks GB, Hui J, Le Souef P, et al. Identification of IL6R and chromosome 11q13.5 as risk loci for asthma. Lancet. 2011;378(9795):1006–14. 3. Bhat SK, Beilin LJ, Robinson M, Burrows S, Mori TA. Contrasting effects of prenatal life stress on blood pressure and body mass index in young adults. J Hypertens. 2015;33(4):711–9. 4. Hollams EM, de Klerk NH, Holt PG, Sly PD. Persistent effects of maternal smoking during pregnancy on lung function and asthma in adolescents. Am J Respir Crit Care Med. 2014;189(4):401–7. 5. Tearne JE, Allen KL, Herbison CE, Lawrence D, Whitehouse AJ, Sawyer MG, et al. The association between prenatal environment and children's mental health trajectories from 2 to 14 years. Eur Child Adolesc Psychiatry. 2015;24(9):1015–24. 1. 6. Hart R, Doherty DA, Frederiksen H, Keelan JA, Hickey M, Sloboda D, et al. The influence of antenatal exposure to phthalates on subsequent female reproductive development in adolescence: a pilot study. Reproduction. 2014;147(4):379–90.
Key reference	Straker L, Mountain J, Jacques A, White S, Smith A, Landau L, Stanley F, Newnham J, Pennell C, Eastwood P. Cohort Profile: The Western Australian Pregnancy Cohort (Raine) Study - Generation 2. Int J Epidemiol. 2017.

Growing Up in New Zealand

Susan Morton

<table>
<tr><td>Name</td><td colspan="3">Growing Up in New Zealand</td><td colspan="2">Abbreviation</td><td>GUINZ</td></tr>
<tr><td>Homepage</td><td colspan="6">www.growingup.co.nz</td></tr>
<tr><td rowspan="2">Recruited number</td><td>Children</td><td>6853</td><td>Mothers</td><td>6823</td><td>Fathers</td><td>4401</td></tr>
<tr><td>Brothers/ sisters</td><td>0</td><td>Grandparents</td><td>0</td><td>Others</td><td>0</td></tr>
<tr><td>Date of enrollment</td><td>Start</td><td colspan="2">2009</td><td>End</td><td colspan="2">ongoing</td></tr>
<tr><td>Principal investigator(s)</td><td colspan="3">Dr Susan Morton</td><td>E-mail</td><td colspan="2">s.morton@auckland.ac.nz</td></tr>
<tr><td>Contact person(s)</td><td colspan="3">Ms Mandy Heathcote</td><td>E-mail</td><td colspan="2">m.heathcote@auckland.ac.nz</td></tr>
<tr><td>Aims</td><td colspan="6">Growing Up in New Zealand is a longitudinal, multidisciplinary pre-birth cohort study designed specifically to understand what shapes developmental trajectories for contemporary New Zealand children growing up in the twenty-first century. The study's explicit objective is to be translational, that is, to provide population-relevant evidence about what influences children's well-being, to inform the evaluation and implementation of cross-sectorial policy initiatives that can improve the health and well-being of all New Zealand children</td></tr>
<tr><td>Public health activities</td><td colspan="6">From the development phase onward, Growing Up in New Zealand has created partnerships with policymakers across multiple sectors to facilitate the relevance of and the translation of the research findings
Policy relevance and utility is a key goal for Growing Up in New Zealand. This is achieved through (1) specific translational objectives and research questions, (2) engagement with policymakers throughout the design phase, and (3) continued and ongoing engagement with policymakers at all steps of data collection and dissemination. This engagement is mediated by the Growing Up in New Zealand Policy Forum, a multi-agency reference group of senior policy advisors representing 16 government agencies including the Ministry of Health. This forum meets several times a year to review data collection plans and data analysis and inform reporting and translation of research and policy outputs. The multi-sector engagement recognizes that improving population health from birth requires engagement beyond health per se.
To date the study has produced over 100 scientific manuscripts detailing children's early development in the NZ context. Additionally several hundred policy-specific outputs (comprehensive reports, select committee submissions, policy briefs, and fast-track outputs to address Ministerial questions) have been developed in partnership with stakeholders to enable translation of the robust scientific outputs to provide evidence for policymakers and communities (outputs available at www.growingup.co.nz)
A Data Access Protocol protects the cohort's privacy and also oversees all data access. Anonymized datasets are made available for all researchers and policy agencies to utilize to undertake policy-relevant research to improve well-being
The team engage with participants regularly via quarterly newsletters, birthday cards for the children, and the website (www.growingup.co.nz). Media opportunities are frequent, and participants are informed of all outputs in advance of public release to recognize the value of their engagement in the study
Study findings are disseminated at stakeholder events and national and international conferences and via policy agencies
Further details are available on the website</td></tr>
<tr><td>Key reference</td><td colspan="6">Morton SM, Atatoa Carr PE, Grant CC, Robinson EM, Bandara DK, Bird A, et al. Cohort profile: growing up in New Zealand. Int J Epidemiol. 2012;42:65–75. https://doi.org/10.1093/ije/dyr206.</td></tr>
</table>

Growing Up in Singapore Towards healthy Outcomes

Yap Seng Chong

Name	Growing Up in Singapore Towards Healthy Outcomes			**Abbreviation**		GUSTO
Homepage	http://gusto.sg					
Recruited number	**Children**	1176	**Mothers**	1247	**Fathers**	820
	Brothers/sisters	–	**Grandparents**	–	**Others**	–
Date of enrollment	**Start**	June 2009		**End**	Sept 2010	
Principal investigator(s)	A/Prof Yap-Seng CHONG			**E-mail**	obgcys@nus.edu.sg	
Contact person(s)	Dr. Shu-E SOH			**E-mail**	paesse@nus.edu.sg	
Aims	To precisely define the critical developmental pathways and mechanisms of the origins of obesity, metabolic disease, and neurodevelopmental disorders that have major public health and economic importance in Asia and globally, with the goal to develop precision medicine approaches (biomarkers and interventions) for children at risk of future noncommunicable diseases					
Public health activities	Our studies have already had major academic and translational impact and attracted significant media attention and policymaker interest. Some examples of the translation of our science into public health activities are highlighted below ***Gestational Diabetes Mellitus*** Gestational diabetes mellitus (GDM) has been found to be much more prevalent than previously thought, affecting up to one in five GUSTO women, with differing frequency for Chinese, Malay, and Indian. The current high-risk approach recommended by local authorities for screening women for GDM misses half the actual cases. Even in the absence of GDM, higher fasting glucose levels can affect infant adiposity and neural development, suggesting that medical observation and evaluation are needed at levels below the formal diagnostic criteria. Following delivery, preliminary analyses showed that women who were diagnosed with GDM during pregnancy had over 11 times the risk of developing type 2 diabetes (11.0%) compared to those who were not diagnosed with GDM (0.7%) within 5 years of the index pregnancy. We submitted a formal report to the Ministry of Health in September 2015, which has already influenced the GDM screening policy in the three public maternity units in Singapore. We will continue to review the GDM diagnostic criteria that are suitable for the local population and work with the Ministry to set up a national GDM registry for long-term follow-up and surveillance ***Maternal Emotional Well-being*** Prior research, as well as our findings in GUSTO, strongly suggests that depression and anxiety in women during pregnancy have important effects on birth outcomes and fetal brain development. A formal report has been submitted to the Ministry of Health in September 2015 to suggest that easy-to-administer screening tools be integrated into routine prenatal and postnatal care across all government and private maternity hospitals to identify women with high levels of depressive or anxiety symptoms embarking on pregnancies as well as in the stressful postnatal period. Women with significant symptoms or risk factors should be followed up with professional support by allied health personnel during pregnancy and continuity of care from hospital to home. Risk factors and social determinants for antenatal and postnatal anxiety and depression should be identified to provide targeted help for high-risk groups ***Antenatal Micronutrient Status*** Our findings, together with the work of the EpiGen Consortium, have led to the Nutritional Intervention Preconception and during Pregnancy to maintain healthy glucosE levels and offspRing health (NiPPeR) clinical trial, which will lead to important new knowledge for the development of better nutrition guidelines for prospective parents, pregnant women, infants, and children					
Key reference	Soh SE, Tint MT, Gluckman PD, Godfrey KM, Rifkin-Graboi A, Chan YH, et al. Cohort profile: growing up in Singapore Towards healthy Outcomes (GUSTO) birth cohort study. Int J Epidemiol. 2014;43(5):1401–9.					

Hokkaido Study on Environment and Children's Health

Reiko Kishi

Name	The Hokkaido study of Environment and Children's Health: Hokkaido Large-Scale Cohort and Sapporo Cohort			**Abbreviation**		The Hokkaido Study
Homepage	http://www.cehs.hokudai.ac.jp/hokkaidostudyen/					
Recruited number Hokkaido / Sapporo cohort	**Children**	20,803/511	**Mothers**	20,926/514	**Fathers**	0/0
	Brothers/ sisters	0/0	**Grandparents**	0/0	**Others**	0/0
Date of enrollment	**Start**	2002		**End**	ongoing	
Principal investigator(s)	Dr. Reiko Kishi			**E-mail**	rkishi@med.hokudai.ac.jp	
Contact person(s)	Dr. Reiko Kishi			**E-mail**	rkishi@med.hokudai.ac.jp	
Aims	The Hokkaido study is an ongoing cohort study that began in 2002. The study consists of two perspective birth cohorts, the Sapporo cohort ($n = 514$) and the Hokkaido large-scale cohort ($n = 20{,}926$). The primary goals of this study are to first examine the potential negative effects of perinatal environmental chemical exposures on birth outcomes, including congenital malformations and growth retardation; second, to evaluate the development of allergies, infectious diseases, and neurodevelopmental disorders and perform longitudinal observations of the children's physical development to clarify the casual relationship between these outcomes and environmental chemicals; and, finally, to identify gene-environment interaction among susceptible population with SNPs and molecular mechanisms via epigenetics.					
Public health activities	The Hokkaido study offers variety of public activities such as website, newsletters, health information, health and developmental consultation with participants, and suggestion for health policy ***Website*** The Hokkaido study maintains a website not only for participants but also for the general public. We introduce our studies and research achievements and announce events for the study participants and citizens (Fig. A.1) ***Newsletter*** The Hokkaido study sends newsletter twice a year which explains research achievement. We also provide information leaflets concerning childcare once a year and announce events for participants ***Booklet for Children*** Children who participate in early period reach 13 years old. In order to convince children themselves of importance of the study, we made a booklet for children. The booklet contains the process of investigation and future plan, with easy-to-understand explanation (Fig. A.2) ***Events*** We organize events for participants to provide research results and health information					

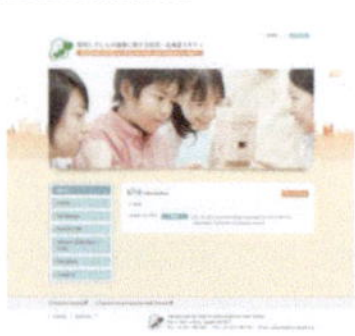

Fig. A.1 Web site

Fig. A.2 Booklet for children

(continued)

Key reference	Kishi et al. The Hokkaido Birth Cohort Study on Environment and Children's Health: cohort profile—updated 2017. Environ Health Prev Med. 2017;22:46. Kishi et al. Ten years of progress in the Hokkaido Birth Cohort Study on Environment and Children's Health: cohort profile—updated 2013. Environ Health Prev Med. 2013;18:429–450. Kishi et al. Cohort profile: the Hokkaido Study on Environment and Children's Health in Japan. Int J Epidemiol. 2011;40:611–8.

Chiba study of Mother and Child Health (C-MACH)

Kenichi Sakurai and Chisato Mori

Name	Chiba study of Mother and Child Health			**Abbreviation**		C-MACH
Homepage	http://cpms.chiba-u.jp/kids/					
Recruited number	**Children**	358	**Mothers**	433	**Fathers**	355
	Brothers/sisters	0	**Grandparents**	0	**Others**	0
Date of enrollment	**Start**	2014		**End**	Ongoing	
Principal investigator(s)	Chisato Mori			**E-mail**	cmori@faculty.chiba-u.jp	
Contact person(s)	Kenichi Sakurai			**E-mail**	sakuraik@faculty.chiba-u.jp	
Aims	Chiba study of Mother and Child Health (C-MACH) should be regarded as a birth cohort study using "omics" analysis, including genome, methylome, metabolome, and metagenome analysis. Environmental factors such as maternal lifestyle and nutritional status, indoor dust, and environmental chemicals including in utero exposure are assessed. The study consists of three hospital-based cohorts in Chiba prefecture and Saitama prefecture, Japan. The aim of C-MACH is to provide a broad-based platform for both present research topics and those that will emerge in the future					

(continued)

(continued)

Public health activities	Chiba study of Mother and Child Health (C-MACH) offers several public activities such as a website and newsletter Website C-MACH maintains a website open to not only participants but also the general public in Japanese (Fig. A.3). We provide information about the aim and methods of C-MACH. We will also provide the results of C-MACH Newsletter C-MACH sends newsletters (Fig. A.4), cards, and gifts to participants to stay in touch. We provide information about child care and results from C-MACH in the newsletters. Newsletters can be read on our website 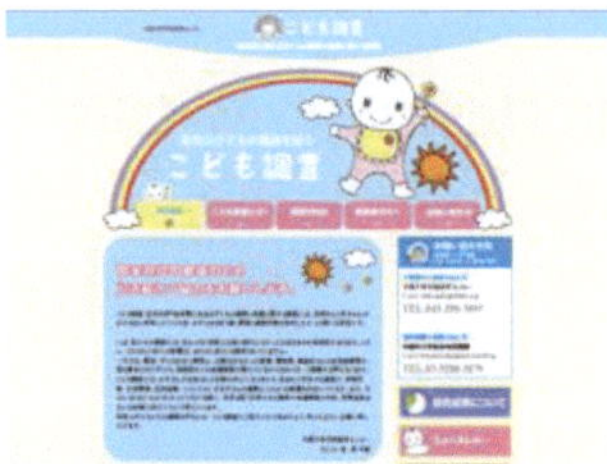 **Fig. A.3** Top page of C-MACH website. 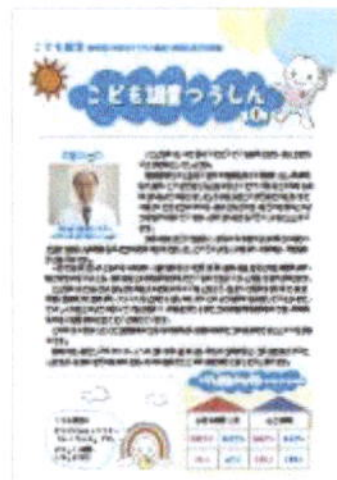 **Fig. A.4** A newsletter of C-MACH. Newsletters are sent to the participants and can be read on our website.
Key reference	Sakurai K, Miyaso H, Eguchi A, Matsuno Y, Yamamoto M, Todaka E, Fukuoka H, Hata A, Mori C. Cohort profile: Chiba study of Mother and Children's Health (C-MACH): cohort study with omics analyses: cohort study with omics analyses. BMJ Open. 2016;6:e010531. https://doi.org/10.1136/bmjopen-2015-010531. Tachibana K, Sakurai K, Watanabe M, Miyaso H, Mori C. Associations between changes in the maternal gut microbiome and differentially methylated regions of diabetes-associated genes in fetuses: a pilot study from the a birth cohort study. J Diabetes Investig (in press).

Hamamatsu Birth Cohort for Mothers and Children (HBC Study)

Kenji Tsuchiya

Name	Hamamatsu Birth Cohort for Mothers and Children		**Abbreviation**		HBC Study
Homepage	http://birthcohorts.net/bch2/?action=show&UserID=146				
Recruited number	**Children**	1258	**Mothers** 1138	**Fathers**	1138
	Brothers/sisters	(82)*	**Grandparents** 0	**Others**	0
Date of enrollment	**Start**	2007	**End**	2011	

(continued)

Principal investigator(s)	Kenji J. Tsuchiya Shu Takagai	**E-mail**	tsuchiya@hama-med.ac.jp takagai@hama-med.ac.jp
Contact person(s)	Kenji J. Tsuchiya Shu Takagai	**E-mail**	tsuchiya@hama-med.ac.jp takagai@hama-med.ac.jp
Aims	The Hamamatsu Birth Cohort for Mothers and Children (HBC Study) is a multidisciplinary birth cohort study investigating the trajectories of neurodevelopmental derailments and abnormalities in a representative sample of Japanese children. Our primary interest is to elucidate trajectories of children who later will be diagnosed as having developmental disorders including autism spectrum disorder, using frequent face-to-face monitoring (e.g. eight times during the first 2 years)		
Public health activities	The Hamamatsu Birth Cohort for Mothers and Children (HBC Study) provides a range of contributions in local health activities as well as in more general, public health terms Collaboration with local government: The HBC Study team has regular discussions over health policies for children in the City of Hamamatsu (population: ca. 810,000), particularly over emerging problems of developmental derailment and developmental disorders. The team sends its staff for regional centres in the City to conduct routine health and developmental checkups of young children and to offer guidance and advice for local health professionals Public awareness activities: The HBC Study team hosts events for World Autism Awareness Day (Fig. A.5) in the City of Hamamatsu, on 2 April of every year	Fig. A.5 Logo for World Autism Awareness Day	
Key reference	1. Takagai S, Tsuchiya KJ, Itoh H, Kanayama N, Mori N, Takei N, on behalf of HBC Study Team. Cohort profile: Hamamatsu Birth Cohort for Mothers and Children (HBC Study). Int J Epidemiol. 2016;45(2):333–42. 2. Nishimura T, Takei N, Tsuchiya KJ, Asano R, Mori N. Identification of neurodevelopmental trajectories in infancy and of risk factors affecting deviant development: a longitudinal birth cohort study. Int J Epidemiol. 2016;45:543–53.		

The Toyama Birth Cohort Study (the Toyama study)

Michikazu Sekine

Name	The Toyama Birth Cohort Study (the Toyama study)		**Abbreviation**		TBCS
Homepage	http://www.med.u-toyama.ac.jp/healpro/toyamast/toyamastindex.html				
Recruited number	**Children**	Approx.10,000	**Mothers**		**Fathers**
	Brothers/sisters		**Grandparents**		**Others**

(continued)

Date of enrollment	**Start**	1992	**End**	
Principal investigator(s)	Michikazu Sekine, MD, MBA		**E-mail**	sekine@med.u-toyama.ac.jp
Contact person(s)	Masaaki Yamada, MD		**E-mail**	masaakit@med.u-toyama.ac.jp
Aims	The Toyama Birth Cohort Study is a prospective cohort study. All of the subjects were born in the periods between April 1989 and March 1990. The initial survey was conducted in 1992 when they were 3 years of age, with follow-up surveys undertaken every 3 years. Information on socioeconomic status, parental and child anthropometric characteristics, lifestyle factors, and physical and mental health measures were collected. The main aim of our study is to identify environmental and lifestyle factors which may influence physical and mental health of children			
Public health activities	Main findings from our study are as follows: (1) parental and lifestyle factors influencing the development of child obesity and poor quality of life (QOL) are parental obesity, skipping breakfast, snacking, physical inactivity, long hours of TV watching, long hours of video game playing, late bedtime, and short sleep hours; short sleep hours in the preschool years was associated with the development of obesity; (2) children who continued to have these risk factors for obesity had the highest risk for the incidence of child obesity, in comparison with those who kept desirable lifestyles; (3) the number of obesity risk factors for children was positively associated with an increased risk for the incidence of child obesity; (4) socioeconomic and family characteristics including family structure, maternal employment status, and maternal obesity were mildly to moderately associated with the obesity risk factors; (5) children's lifestyle factors in the preschool years were associated with future lifestyle factors. The strategy for preventing obesity should be focused on socioeconomic and family characteristics and children's lifestyle factors from their preschool years **Newsletter:** We have published newsletters for the subjects and their parents **Report:** We have published reports for schools, educational committees, public health centers, and local government **Website:** The main findings from our study are shown in our website. Individuals can freely use figures and tables in the website for various purposes **Newspapers and Magazines:** The findings from our study have often appeared in newspapers and magazines **Health Education:** We have often provided health education for children and their parents on the basis of the findings from our study **Human Resource Development:** We have had lectures and seminars for public health nurses, school nurses, teachers, and members of Educational Committee **Collaboration for Child Health Research:** We have provided know-hows to conduct child health research (e.g., the Japan Environment and Children's Study) **Policy Recommendations:** The study results have often been used for health policy through, for example, recommendations by the Science Council of Japan			
Key reference	2. Sekine M, Yamagami T, Handa K, et al. A dose-response relationship between short sleeping hours and childhood obesity: results from the Toyama birth cohort study. Child Care Health Dev. 2002;28:163–70. 3. Sekine M, Yamagami T, Kagamimori S. Lifestyle and childhood obesity: results from the Toyama birth cohort study. Pediatr Cardiol Cardiac Surg. 2008;24:589–97 (a review paper in Japanese). 4. Sekine M. Eating and sleep: social determinants of lifestyle factors and their correlations. In: Negayama K, Toyama N, Kawahara N, editors. Reshaping children's development of eating: from multi-disciplinary views. Tokyo: University of Tokyo Press; 2013. p.197–210 (a book chapter in Japanese).			

Project Koshu

Zentaro Yamagata

<table>
<tr><td>Name</td><td colspan="3">Project Koshu</td><td>Abbreviation</td><td colspan="2">N/A</td></tr>
<tr><td>Homepage</td><td colspan="6">N/A</td></tr>
<tr><td rowspan="2">Recruited number</td><td>Children</td><td>5000</td><td>Mothers</td><td>5000</td><td>Fathers</td><td>N/A</td></tr>
<tr><td>Brothers/sisters</td><td>N/A</td><td>Grandparents</td><td>N/A</td><td>Others</td><td>N/A</td></tr>
<tr><td>Date of enrollment</td><td>Start</td><td colspan="2">1988</td><td>End</td><td colspan="2">Ongoing</td></tr>
<tr><td>Principal investigator(s)</td><td colspan="3">Prof. Zentaro Yamagata</td><td>E-mail</td><td colspan="2">zenymgt@yamanashi.ac.jp</td></tr>
<tr><td>Contact person(s)</td><td colspan="3">Prof. Zentaro Yamagata</td><td>E-mail</td><td colspan="2">zenymgt@yamanashi.ac.jp</td></tr>
<tr><td>Aims</td><td colspan="6">The purpose of the study was to describe the current status of maternal and child health in the Koshu City. For example, a trend of maternal smoking during pregnancy was previously reported. Then, after accumulating the data from each year, longitudinal datasets were created to examine the association between exposures in fetal and infant periods, such as maternal smoking during pregnancy or childhood sleep duration, and childhood growth and development. Thus, depending on the research question, various cohorts were able to be established</td></tr>
<tr><td>Public health activities</td><td colspan="6">Leaflets
Based on the results from Project Koshu, public health nurses of Koshu administration office and members of the Department of Health Sciences produced the leaflets which aimed to prevent not only maternal smoking and alcohol consumption during pregnancy but also passive smoking among pregnant women. These leaflets are distributed to women who register their pregnancy with the administration office (Fig. A.6)
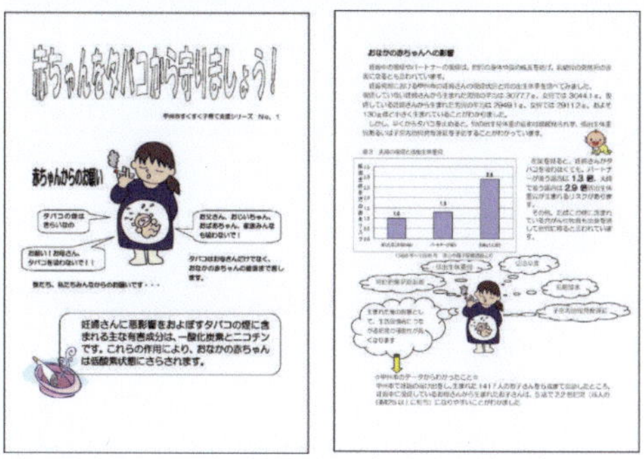

Fig. A.6 Leaflet based on the results from Project Koshu
Suggestion for Health Policy
Some results from the study were used as a baseline data of health policy in Koshu City. These results were also provided the longitudinal assessment of the policy</td></tr>
<tr><td>Key reference</td><td colspan="6">Kohta Suzuki:Longitudinal analyses of childhood growth: evidence from Project Koshu. J Epidemiol. 2015;25(1):2–7.</td></tr>
</table>

Appendix B: Birth Cohorts and Consortia in the World

Symbol	Full name	URL
Consortia and networks		
BiCCA	Birth Cohort Consortium of Asia	http://www.bicca.org/
Birthcohots.net	Birthcohots.net	http://www.birthcohorts.net/
CHARGE	Cohorts for Heart and Aging Research in Genomic Epidemiology	http://www.chargeconsortium.com/
CHICOS	Developing a Child Cohort Research Strategy for Europe	http://www.chicosproject.eu/the-project/
CLOSER	Cohort and Longitudinal Studies Enhancement Resources	https://www.closer.ac.uk/
EAGLE	EArly Genetics and Lifecourse Epidemiology Consortium	https://www.wikigenes.org/e/art/e/348.html
Early Nutrition	Long-term Effects of Early Nutrition on Later Health	http://www.project-earlynutrition.eu/eneu/
EGG	Early Growth Genetics Consortium	https://egg-consortium.org/
ENRIECO	Environmental Health Risks in European Birth Cohorts	http://www.enrieco.org/
EpiGen	EpiGen Global Research Consortium	http://www.epigengrc.com/
Intergrowth-21th	International Fetal and Newborn Growth Consortium	http://www.intergrowth21.org.uk/
MeDALL	Mechanisms of the Development of Allergy	http://www.u4network.eu/index.php/network/projects/273-medall-mechanisms-of-the-development-of-allergy
PACE	Pregnancy And Childhood Epigenetics	https://www.niehs.nih.gov/research/atniehs/labs/epi/pi/genetics/pace/index.cfm

(continued)

F. Sata et al. (eds.), *Pre-emptive Medicine: Public Health Aspects of Developmental Origins of Health and Disease*, Current Topics in Environmental Health and Preventive Medicine, https://doi.org/10.1007/978-981-13-2194-8

Symbol	Full name	URL
Birth cohorts		
ABCB	Aarhus Birth Cohort Biobank	http://fetotox.au.dk/the-fetotox-birth-cohorts/aarhus-birth-cohort-biobank-abcb/
ABCD	Amsterdam Born Children and their Development	http://abcd-studie.nl/
ABIS	All Babies in Southeast Sweden	http://www.abis-studien.se/hem/english-11100423
ALSPAC	Avon Longitudinal Study of Parents and Children	http://www.bristol.ac.uk/alspac/
ArcRisk	Arctic Health Risks: Impacts on health in the Arctic and Europe owing to climate-induced changes in contaminant cycling	http://www.oulu.fi/arctichealth/arcrisk
BAMSE	Stockholm Children Allergy and Environmental Prospective Birth Cohort Study	http://ki.se/en/imm/bamse-project
BASELINE	Babies After SCOPE: Evaluating the Longitudinal Impact using Neurological and Nutritional Endpoints	http://www.infantcentre.ie/our-research/research-studies/baseline
BCS70	1970 British Cohort Study	https://cls.ucl.ac.uk/clsstudies/1970-british-cohortstudy/
BiB	Born in Bradford	https://borninbradford.nhs.uk/
BienHoa study	BienHoa Dioxin Cohort study	–
BILD	Bern-Basel Infant Lung Development Cohort	http://www.bild-cohort.ch/en/
Birth Cohort Study in Mongolia	Birth Cohort Study in Mongolia-Towards Solving Global Problems in the Maternal and Child Health	–
BirThree Cohort Study	Tohoku Medical Megabank Project Birth and Three-Generation Cohort Study	http://www.megabank.tohoku.ac.jp/english/about/member/group05/
CATSS	Child and Adolescent Twin Study in Sweden	http://ki.se/en/meb/the-child-and-adolescent-twin-study-in-sweden-catss
CCC2000	Copenhagen Child Cohort	https://www.regionh.dk/CCC2000/Sider/default.aspx
CHAMACOS	Center for Health Assessment of Mothers and Children of Salinas	https://cerch.berkeley.edu/research-programs/chamacos-study
CHECK	Children's Health and Environmental Chemicals in Korea	–
CHEF	Children's Health and the Environment in the Faroes	http://www.chef-project.dk/
CHOP (EU)	Childhood Obesity – Early Programming by Infant Nutrition	http://www.metabolic-programming.org/obesity/

(continued)

Symbol	Full name	URL
CHOP (USA)	Children's Hospital of Philadelphia	http://www.chop.edu/
CHS	Children's Health Study	https://healthstudy.usc.edu/
CLHNS	Cebu Longitudinal Health and Nutrition Survey	http://www.cpc.unc.edu/projects/cebu
COCOA	Cohort for Childhood Origin of Asthma and allergic diseases	–
Co.N.ER	Bologna birth cohort	–
COSPAC	Copenhagen Prospective Studies on Asthma in Childhood	http://copsac.com/
DaDoCiV	Dioxin and Development of Children in Vietnam	–
DaNang	DaNang Dioxin Cohort study	–
DARC	Danish Allergy Research Centre	–
DNBC	Danish National Birth Cohort	https://www.ssi.dk/English/RandD/Research%20areas/Epidemiology/DNBC/
DONALD	DOrtmund Nutritional and Anthropometric Longitudinally Designed Studies	https://www.ernaehrungsepidemiologie.uni-bonn.de/forschung/donald-1
ECHO Program	Environmental influences on Child Health Outcomes Program	https://www.nih.gov/echo
EDC study	Environment and Development of Children Study	–
EDEN	Étude des Déterminants pré et postnatals du développement et de la santé de l'Enfant	http://eden.vjf.inserm.fr/index.php/fr/
EFSOCH	Exeter Family Study of Childhood Health	http://www.diabetesgenes.org/content/exeter-family-study-childhood-health
EHL	Growing up in Wales: The Environments for Healthy Living study	–
ELFE	Étude Longitudinale Française depuis l'Enfance	http://www.elfe-france.fr/
ERF	Erasmus Rucphen Family study	–
EPIC	European Prospective Investigation into Cancer	http://epic.iarc.fr/
FCOU	Family and Children of Ukraine	http://globalhealth.uic.edu/research/ongoing-research-projects/family-and-children-of-ukraine
FLEHS	Flemish Environment and Health Survey	–
G21	Generation XXI	http://projectogeracaoxxi-contactos.blogspot.jp/

Symbol	Full name	URL
GALA	Genes-environments and Admixture in Latino Americans	https://pharm.ucsf.edu/gala
GASPII	Genetica e Ambiente: Studio Prospettico dell'Infanzia in Italia	–
GECKO	Groningen Expert Center for Kids with Obesity	https://www.umcg.nl/NL/Zorg/Volwassenen/deelname_wetenschappelijk_onderzoek/GECKO%20Drenthe%20-%20Overgewicht%20bij%20kinderen/Paginas/default.aspx
Generation R	Generation R	https://www.generationr.nl/
GMS	Gateshead Millennium Study	http://research.ncl.ac.uk/gms/
GUS	Growing Up in Scotland	http://growingupinscotland.org.uk/
GINIplus	German Infant Study on the influence of Nutrition Intervention	http://www.ginistudie.de/
GOYA	Genomics of Overweight Young Adults	–
GUSTO	Growing up in Singapore Towards Health Outcomes	http://www.gusto.sg/
HBC study	Hamamatsu Birth Cohort for Mothers and Children	http://rccmd.org/modules/research/index.php?content_id=4
HBCS	Helsinki Birth Cohort Study	https://www.thl.fi/fi/web/thlfi-en/research-and-expertwork/projects-and-programmes/helsinki-birth-cohort-study-hbcs-idefix
HCS	Hertfordshire Cohort Study	https://www.mrc.soton.ac.uk/herts/
HHf2	Healthy Habits for two	–
Hokkaido Study	Hokkaido Study on Environment and Children's Health	https://www.cehs.hokudai.ac.jp/hokkaidostudyen/
HRBC	Harvard Reproductive and Birth Cohort	–
HUMIS	Norwegian Human Milk Study	https://www.fhi.no/en/projects/HUMIS/
INMA Project	INMA-Environment and Childhood Project	http://www.proyectoinma.org/en_index.html
INUENDO	Human Fertility at Risk from Biopersistent Organochlorines in the Environments	–
Isle of Wight Birth Cohort	Isle of Wight Birth Cohort	http://www.allergyresearch.org.uk/studies/birth-cohort/
IVAAQ	Greenland Inuit child cohort	–
JECS	Japan Environment and Children's Study	http://www.env.go.jp/en/chemi/hs/jecs/

(continued)

Symbol	Full name	URL
KANC	Kaunas Cohort	–
KCHS	Kalutara Children's Health Study	–
KOALA	KOALA Birth Cohort Study	https://www.koala-study.nl/koala-birth-cohort-study
Ko-CHENS	Korean Children's Environmental Health Study	http://cms.ewha.ac.kr/user/indexSub.action?codyMenuSeq=3315490&siteId=ewhamedeng
Koshu Project	Koshu Project	http://www.med.yamanashi.ac.jp/medicine/birthcohort/study/summary/koshuProject.html
LISA	Influence of life-style factors on the development of the immune system and allergies in East and West Germany	https://www.helmholtzmuenchen.de/epi/research/research-groups/allergicdisease-epidemiology/projects/lisa/index.html
LRC	Leicester & Rutland Cohort Studies	https://www.leicestercohorts.org/index.php?id=2578
LWBC	Laizhou Wan Birth Cohort	–
MAS 5	Cities birth cohort	–
MAS-90	Multizentrische Allergie Studie	https://www.aeda.de/presse/pressearchiv/einzelansicht/?tx_ttnews%5Btt_news%5D=222&cHash=3d0c9ba5f010418ce59c4550cd793c4d
MCS	Millennium Cohort Study	http://www.cls.ioe.ac.uk/page.aspx?sitesectionid=851
MEFAB	Maastricht Essential Fatty Acid Birth	http://www.mefab.org/
MISC	Mother Infant Study Cohort	–
MoBa	Norwegian Mother and Child Cohort	https://www.fhi.no/en/studies/moba/
MOCEH	Mothers and Children's Environmental Health study	https://www.niehs.nih.gov/research/programs/geh/partnerships/network/cohorts/moceh/index.cfm
NCCGP	North Cumbria Community Genetics Projects	http://research.ncl.ac.uk/plerg/Research/Genetic%20Epidemiology/NCCGP.htm
NCDS	1958 National Child Development Study (British Birth Cohort)	https://cls.ucl.ac.uk/clsstudies/1958-national-childdevelopment-study/
Nepali	Nepali Birth Cohort Study in Chitwan Valley	–
NEST	Newborn Epigenetics Study	https://sites.duke.edu/nest/
NFBC	Northern Finland Birth Cohorts	http://www.oulu.fi/nfbc/

Symbol	Full name	URL
NFCS	Norway Facial Clefts Study	https://www.niehs.nih.gov/research/atniehs/labs/epi/studies/ncl/index.cfm
NINFEA	Nascita e INFanzia: gli Effetti dell'Ambiente	http://www.progettoninfea.it
NiPPeR	Nutritional Intervention Preconception and During Pregnancy to Maintain Healthy Glucose Metabolism and Offspring Health	https://www.nipperstudy.com/about-nipper
NJMUBC	Nanjing Medical University Birth Cohort	–
NorFlu	Norwegian Influenza Cohort Study	–
NTR	Netherlands Twin Registry	http://fastfacts.nl/en/content/netherlands-twin-register
Newcastle Thousand Families Study	Newcastle Thousand Families Study	http://research.ncl.ac.uk/plerg/Research/1000F/1000_home.htm
NSHD/1946BC	MRC National Survey of Health and Development Cohort/1946 Birth Cohort	http://www.nshd.mrc.ac.uk/
Odense Child Cohort	Odense Child Cohort	http://subsites.odense.dk/subsites2/odensebornekohorte
ORCADES	Orkney Complex Disease Study	https://www.ed.ac.uk/viking/about-us/orcades
Origins Project	Origins Project	https://originsproject.telethonkids.org.au/
PANIC	Physical Activity and Nutrition in Children	–
PCB Cohort	Early Childhood Development and PCB exposures in Slovakia	http://slovakchildren.ucdavis.edu/
PÉLAGIE	Endocrine disruptors: Longitudinal study on pregnancy abnormalities, infertility, and childhood	–
PIAMA	Prevention and Incidence of Asthma and Mite Allergy	http://piama.iras.uu.nl/index-en.php
Piccolipiù	Piccolipiù	http://www.piccolipiu.it
Predict Study	Rotterdam Periconceptional Cohort Study	–
PRIDE Study	PRegnancy and Infant DEvelopment Study	https://pridestudy.nl/index.html
Project VIVA	Project VIVA: A Study of Health for The Next Generation	https://www.hms.harvard.edu/viva/
PSKC	Panel Study on Korean Children	http://panel.kicce.re.kr/eng/
RAINE	Western Australian Pregnancy Cohort	https://www.rainestudy.org.au/
REPRO_PL	Polish Mother and Child Cohort Study	http://repropl.com/
RHEA	The Rhea Mother-Child Study in Crete	http://www.rhea.gr/
SBC	Shanghai Birth Cohort	https://www.maelstrom-research.org/mica/individual-study/sbc
SEATON	Study of eczema and asthma to observe the effects of nutrition	https://www.abdn.ac.uk/seatonstudy/science/

(continued)

Symbol	Full name	URL
SEED	Study to Explore Early Development	https://www.cdc.gov/ncbddd/autism/seed.html
SNiP	Survey of Neonates in Pomerania	https://www.ernaehrungs-umschau.de/print-artikel/13-09-2013-snip-survey-of-neonates-in-pomerania-greifswalder-neugeborenenstudie-snip-wird-fortgesetzt/
STRIP	Special Turku Coronary Risk Factor Intervention Project	http://stripstudy.utu.fi/english.html
SWS	Southampton Women's Survey	https://www.mrc.soton.ac.uk/sws/
TBPS	Taiwan Birth Panel Study	http://www.rhlab.org/tbps.html
TCHAD	Twin Study of Child and Adolescent Development	http://ki.se/en/meb/twin-study-of-child-and-adolescent-development-tchad
TEC	Taiwan Early-Life Cohort	–
TEDS	Twins Early Development Study	http://www.teds.ac.uk/
TMICS	Taiwan Maternal and Infant Cohort Study	–
Toyama Study	Toyama Study	http://www.med.u-toyama.ac.jp/healpro/toyamast/toyamastindex.html
TSCD	Tohoku Study of Child Development	–
UGAAR Study	Ulaanbaatar Gestation and Air Pollution Research Study	http://www.sfu.ca/ugaar/home_eng.html
UKHLS	Understanding Society: The UK Household Longitudinal Study	https://www.understandingsociety.ac.uk/
USM pregnancy cohort	Universiti Sains Malaysia Pregnancy Cohort Study	–
WHISTLER	Wheezing Illnesses Study in LEidsche Rijn	http://www.lrgp.nl/
YFS	Young Finns Study	http://youngfinnsstudy.utu.fi/

MIX
Papier aus verantwortungsvollen Quellen
Paper from responsible sources
FSC® C105338

If you have any concerns about our products,
you can contact us on
ProductSafety@springernature.com

In case Publisher is established outside the EU,
the EU authorized representative is:
Springer Nature Customer Service Center GmbH
Europaplatz 3, 69115 Heidelberg, Germany

Printed by Libri Plureos GmbH
in Hamburg, Germany